the little black book of *sex* positions

the little black book of *sex* positions

Jennifer Baritchi and Dan Baritchi

Images by
FlirtynFun Photography

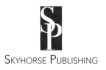

SKYHORSE PUBLISHING

Skyhorse Publishing books may be purchased in bulk at special discounts for sales promotion, corporate gifts, fund-raising, or educational purposes. Special editions can also be created to specifications. For details, contact the Special Sales Department, Skyhorse Publishing, 307 West 36th Street, 11th Floor, New York, NY 10018 or info@skyhorsepublishing.com.

Skyhorse® and Skyhorse Publishing® are registered trademarks of Skyhorse Publishing, Inc.®, a Delaware corporation.

Visit our website at www.skyhorsepublishing.com.

11 10 9 8

Images by FlirtynFun Photography

Library of Congress Cataloging-in-Publication Data is available on file.

ISBN: 978-1-62087-611-4

Printed in China

contents

contents

introduction

This book is about better sex and trying new things including new positions, new places, new games, new props, and new ideas, all in the name of experiencing more pleasure together as a couple. We hope you will dive into this book with an open mind, open heart, and open mouths and legs!

There are three things that can make sex better in every relationship:

1. Setting the mood

2. Committing to better foreplay

3. Agreeing that everyone gets to have an orgasm

There are certain "bedroom products" we believe every couple should own that can dramatically help with these three things. This is where having an open mind comes into play. On our website, AskDanandJennifer.com, we often receive comments such as, "Our sex life is great. We don't need any help," or "Why would we want to use bedroom products?" Well, here's why:

• Because trying new things is fun. We could all use a little more fun and adventure in our lives.

• Because various bedroom products provide a very distinct and unique type of pleasure, which could enrich your sex life as a couple.

• Because both you and your partner have the right to as much pleasure as you can possibly stand.

With all that in mind, here are the top seven bedroom products every couple should own:

1. candles and massage oils

Candles can totally change the mood of a room. They create a warm and romantic environment—just make sure to place them well out of reach. You wouldn't want to accidentally knock one over or catch the bed sheets on fire! Massage oils take the mood from rushed to relaxed and sensual. Keep a good stock of both of these and learn how to give a good, erotic massage.

2. a good lubricant

Every couple should at least have a good water based "lube," and many should have a good silicon lube (or combination lube) for water play. I don't care how wet your partner is, at some point the sex will become less comfortable for her. At that point, she's less likely to orgasm and more likely to just want to get it over with. This is especially true when sex lasts more than fifteen minutes. A woman's body can only keep up for so long! If you've never tried lube, it's time. Just do it! You will never go back . . .

3. clitoral vibrator

Sex toys are a touchy topic for many couples. Men are intimidated because there's no way that their tongue can do what a clitoral vibrator can do for a woman's clitoris. Women for some odd reason feel like they are inadequate if they need a little extra stimulation. We're calling BS on both of these! A clitoral vibrator is a great addition to many of the sex positions that follow—especially for women who love clitoral stimulation.

4. rabbit vibrator

Every girl needs a good rabbit vibrator for two reasons: 1) it helps women get warmed up and really turned on during foreplay, and 2) many women are not able to reach orgasm through vaginal intercourse. Guess what? A rabbit can provide vaginal and clitoral stimulation at the same time. Take some of the pressure off of him and get a good rabbit!

5. male masturbator

Okay boys, if you've never tried a good male masturbator, you are in for a real treat. For those of you who are saying, "I've got my hand. I don't need anything else," you've obviously never tried one of these. Our challenge to you: Try it! You just may like it.

6. liberator wedge

Some of the sex positions that follow can be a little challenging to get into. A wedge will really help. Some of the sex positions that follow do not have a good angle for g-spot stimulation. A wedge will really help. Some of the sex positions that follow do not work for a man with a shorter penis. A wedge will really help. Some of the sex positions that follow . . . You get the idea. A wedge is better than a pillow because it's firmer, and the shape is design to improve "angles of penetration" to make good sex even better.

7. blindfold and silk ties

Even if you're not into the whole "Fifty Shades" scene, you still need at least these two items. Even just a little sensory deprivation caused by a blindfold can awaken all of the other senses! When we can't see, we are force to feel, smell, and listen better. Silk ties are incredible not only because they feel incredible on the skin, but by having our limbs restrained during sex, we have to focus on what our partner is doing to us rather than what we're going to do next. It forces us to turn our brains off and give into the passion of the moment.

Now, off with the clothes and on with the show . . .

chapter 1: missionary sex positions

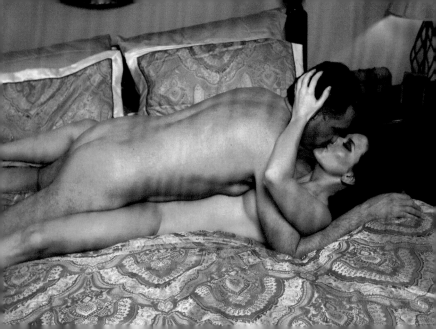

missionary

The "chicken soup" of sex positions, the Missionary is an old favorite enjoyed by many couples. In fact, it's probably the first position you ever tried and might still be your go-to sex position when you just want to experience something familiar. Both partners enjoy this sex position!

HOW TO DO IT The Missionary position is often also called "man on top" and rightly so. The male partner assumes the dominant position on top of the woman, who is lying on her back. Her legs are spread enough so that her lover can thrust, but they're not raised up or resting on his shoulders. While she can thrust some, the primary work done here is by the man.

WHERE TO DO IT The sofa, bed, and floor are all great locations for this position.

PROPS YOU'LL NEED A pillow under her lower back can help support her hips and tilt her pelvis so that penetration is more comfortable and pleasurable.

DIFFICULTY LEVEL ★☆☆☆☆

HER O-METER ★☆☆☆☆ She gets almost nothing physically out of the Missionary position, unless she's already very turned on from a lot of foreplay. It's just not the optimal position for either clitoral or internal stimulation.

HIS O-METER ★★★☆ He fares much better in the Missionary position than she does, simply because he can control the speed and depth of penetration, and he is able to orgasm how and when he wants to. For some guys, however, the Missionary can be little better than getting it on with a blow up doll if their partners are just not that into it.

MAKE IT HOTTER . . . Leave the lights on and gaze into each other's eyes. This type of intimacy is totally hot and allows both partners to fully connect emotionally, which is not always so easy to do!

butterfly

A variation on the standard Missionary, the Butterfly is easy to do yet very satisfying for both male and female partners. There isn't quite as much eye contact here, but the female partner is still positioned in such a way that her lover can stimulate her nipples and clitoris with his hands.

HOW TO DO IT The Butterfly is a much easier version of the Bridge (see page 161). The male partner is in the exact same position actually, which is on his knees, in between his partner's legs. However, instead of arching her back up off the floor, the female partner will support herself on a flat surface that is raised. It's easiest to achieve this position on a bed. The female partner will lie on the bed with her pelvis at the edge of the bed and her feet flat on the floor. If the bed is very high, the male partner can stand, but a lower bed will work better if the male partner would rather be on his knees. He can hold on to her hips for leverage and more control with thrusting. This position is much better for the female partner than the Bridge because it allows her to relax and use something else to support her weight, giving her a better opportunity to actually enjoy it.

WHERE TO DO IT The edge of a low bed or futon works best for this one.

PROPS YOU'LL NEED None.

DIFFICULTY LEVEL ★★★★

HER O-METER ★★★★★ This position is actually fairly comfortable for her and allows her to experience everything more fully. The g-spot penetration is fair here, while the penile clitoral stimulation isn't superb.

HIS O-METER ★★★★★ This sex position is comfortable for him as well, but it's not as exotic as he'd like it to be. He does have control over his orgasm here, but it's just not as exciting for him as the Bridge.

MAKE IT HOTTER . . . A vibrator on her clitoris is the perfect way to give her more pleasure, and if she's enjoying it more, so is he. She can hold the vibrator or he can—both are fun ways to put a twist on this sex position!

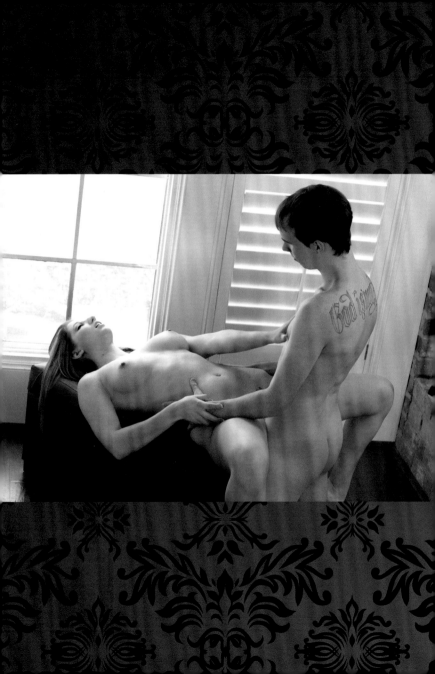

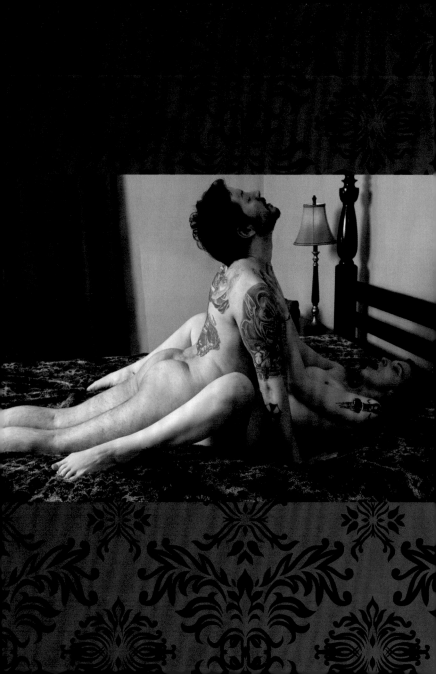

coital alignment technique

The Coital Alignment Technique can be used to increase a woman's chances of orgasm in the Missionary sex position.

HOW TO DO IT Assume the traditional Missionary sex position. The male partner will shift up slightly, while the female partner will shift her hips down slightly, allowing her clitoris and pubic bone to come into contact with the shaft of his penis and his pubic bone.

Since he's not thrusting in and out per se, he's going to be using more of an up-and-down grinding motion. She's going to do her best to grind against him in the same way, keeping her clitoris pressed up against him to receive the stimulation the grinding motion causes. This move actually takes some practice to really get the hang of, but it's totally worth it when she gets to have an amazing orgasm with him on top.

WHERE TO DO IT The bed is best for the Coital Alignment Technique.

PROPS YOU'LL NEED A pillow under her lower back can help angle her pelvis in such a way that it's easier for her to grind against the shaft of his penis and pubic bone.

DIFFICULTY LEVEL ★★★☆☆

HER O-METER ★★★★☆ With the Coital Alignment Technique, she can feel dominated by her guy and get off at the same time.

HIS O-METER ★★★☆☆ The Coital Alignment Technique isn't quite as good for him as it is for her, but he's having sex so, hey, it's all good, right?

MAKE IT HOTTER . . . Gaze deeply into each other's eyes and use this opportunity to connect emotionally as well as physically. When you get good at the Coital Alignment Technique, you can easily use it to achieve simultaneous orgasm!

cowboy

If you can imagine the Cowgirl sex position (see page 38) but with the man on top, you'll have the Cowboy. It's a fun twist on the Missionary, or "him on top" sex!

HOW TO DO IT   The female partner lies on her back with her legs pressed together, as if she were in the traditional Missionary sex position. Her partner will then straddle her with each leg on either side of her to penetrate. He's sitting straight up, "cowboy" style. He's not used to thrusting like this, so it may take some time for him to get the hang of it.

WHERE TO DO IT   A flat surface such as the bed, sofa, or floor is best for the Cowboy sex position. This can be a fun one to do outdoors while camping or doing something else rugged or outdoorsy.

PROPS YOU'LL NEED   Depending on where you do it, she may want a pillow or two under her head, or you may want to spread a blanket out first.

DIFFICULTY LEVEL ★★★☆☆

HER O-METER ★☆☆☆☆   Because he is sitting straight up, it pretty much nixes any hope of constant clitoral contact for her. She does enjoy watching him go at it though, and the g-spot stimulation isn't too shabby either.

HIS O-METER ★★★☆☆   He likes being in control in the Cowboy sex position, but he may think it is too much like the girl on top position, so he may not want to try it. Because her legs aren't spread too far apart, the penetration is nice and tight even though it's not as deep as it is in other sex positions.

MAKE IT HOTTER . . . She may be able to reach down and stimulate her clitoris in the Cowboy sex position, allowing her to receive more pleasure here. However, a hands-free clitoral vibrator that can be worn by her is a fun addition that will heat this sex position up for sure!

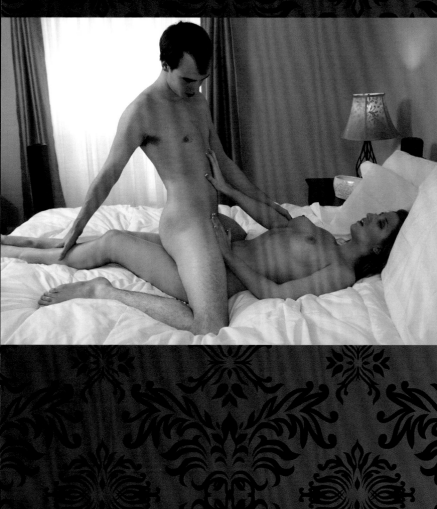

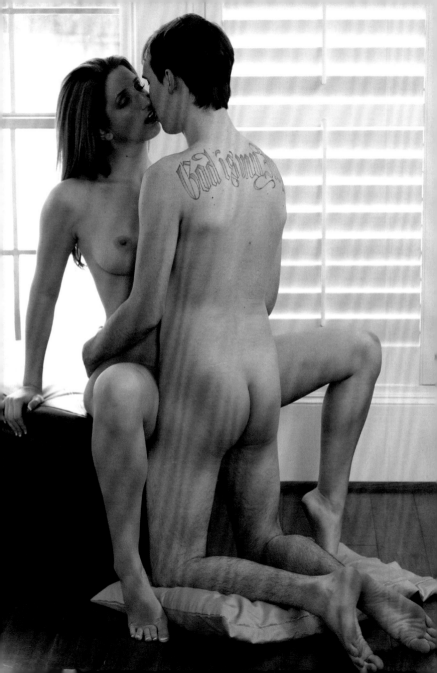

delight

A variation on the Missionary, the Delight is simple but both intimate and erotic. It's a perfect sex position to use if you want lots of eye contact, but it's also great if you want to get kinky and watch the action down below. You definitely want to try this one, and use it again and again!

HOW TO DO IT This is an exceptionally easy sex position to master and is highly arousing and satisfying for both partners. The female partner simply sits on a bed or chair with her legs spread and her feet flat on the floor. The male partner gets on his knees and aligns his pelvis in between her legs for thrusting. It's simple, but both partners get an exceptional amount of pleasure from the Delight!

WHERE TO DO IT The sofa, edge of a low bed, or chair is perfect for this position.

PROPS YOU'LL NEED A soft blanket or pillow for his knees will make this position more comfortable for him.

DIFFICULTY LEVEL ★★★★★

HER O-METER ★★★★★ While this sex position allows for a fair amount of clitoral and g-spot stimulation, that's not what a woman is going to like best about the Delight. Since she is face to face with her partner, she is going to get a lot of emotional satisfaction here. It's a very intimate position, which will definitely be right up her alley.

HIS O-METER ★★★★★ A man will like any position that a woman likes, and, let's face it, guys get pleasure from almost every sex position because of the way a man derives pleasure from sex. It's not as difficult to please a man as it is a woman. This isn't one of the sex positions that will totally *wow* him though.

MAKE IT HOTTER . . . For even hotter intimacy, she can lean forward and cuddle against his chest. Or, if she wants to entice her man, she can lean back and allow him to play with her nipples or massage her clitoris.

drill

Feel every inch of your partner during sex with the intimate but still naughty Drill! It's a sexy twist on the standard Missionary, and allows for super deep penetration.

HOW TO DO IT The main difference between the Drill and the Deck Chair (see page 166) is that instead of raising her legs up where her knees bend at a ninety-degree angle, the female partner wraps her legs around her partner's hips and rests her ankles against his back. This position provides more physical intimacy than the Deck Chair or even the Missionary, because the position of her legs allows for only minimal separation of skin contact. Women, enjoy feeling every inch of your partner with this sex position!

WHERE TO DO IT This versatile position can be done just about anywhere like the sofa, bed, and even the floor.

PROPS YOU'LL NEED Any sex position where the female partner is on her back can be made more comfortable with a pillow under her lower back.

DIFFICULTY LEVEL ★★★★★

HER O-METER ★★★★★ She can keep herself pressed up against him and use her legs muscles to grind her pelvis against her partner's. This provides for awesome clitoral stimulation! Combined with deep penetration, a blended orgasm is definitely possible in this sex position.

HIS O-METER ★★★★★ Because he is on his knees instead of holding up the majority of his own weight with his arms, he can focus more on pleasure than mechanics. This is often a more natural sex position for men than the Missionary.

MAKE IT HOTTER . . . Synchronize your movements so that you're always moving together. Leave the lights on and make deep, sensual eye contact. Go slow and enjoy every sensation and every moment. Your orgasm will be incredible!

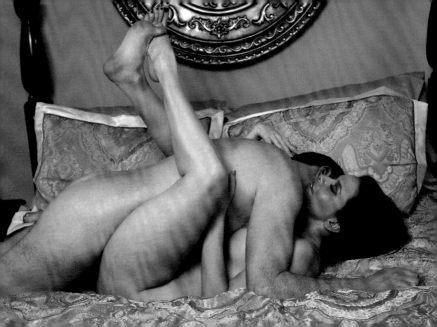

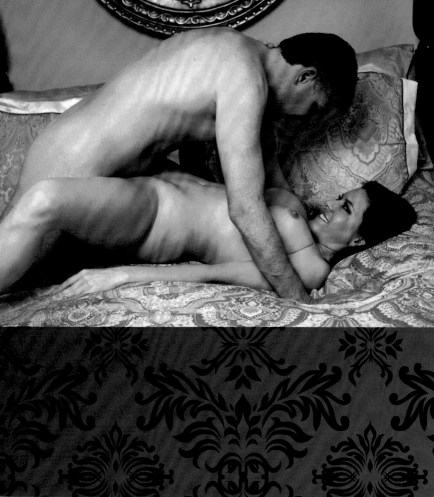

meet 'n' greet

The Meet 'n' Greet puts the thrusting responsibility on the female partner, although she is still on the bottom as in the traditional Missionary position. Instead of him thrusting down into her, she is pushing her pelvis up towards him and doing a majority of the movement. So hot!

HOW TO DO IT Just as in the traditional Missionary position, the male partner is on top and the female partner is underneath him with her legs spread on either side of her lover's hips. He is resting his weight on his knees and his hands, which are on either side of her torso. However, instead of him moving down to thrust into her, she is going to raise her hips again and again to meet him. This requires a good bit of space between both partners, so he will need to prop his torso all the way up on his hands, almost as though he's in the Doggy Style position.

WHERE TO DO IT This position can be done on the sofa, back seat of the car, floor, bed, and anywhere else you would use the Missionary position.

PROPS YOU'LL NEED He may be more comfortable with a pillow under his knees if you're using the Meet 'n' Greet on a hard surface, such as the floor.

DIFFICULTY LEVEL ★☆☆☆☆

HER O-METER ★★★☆☆ Although she has a better chance of grinding her clitoris against him since she's in control in the Meet 'n' Greet, a woman isn't used to thrusting and may tire out quickly. She may not be able to keep this going for very long if she's not fit or strong.

HIS O-METER ★★★★☆ He digs the Meet 'n' Greet sex position because he gets to watch her thrust up towards him instead of the other way around. It's a welcome change of pace, and he totally loves the idea of her being so hot and turned on that she's got to grind against him!

MAKE IT HOTTER . . . It's a great opportunity for her to show him just how eager she is and to really put on a show for him, by playing with her breasts and clitoris while he watches in ecstasy.

missionary reversed

The Missionary Reversed sex position is a fun one to try if his penis is fairly flexible and he's up for something a little more exotic.

HOW TO DO IT The female partner will lie flat on her back with her legs slightly spread. Her partner will then position himself on top of her, but he will be facing her feet instead of her head. His legs will also be spread enough so that they can rest on his lover's shoulders or on either side of her head. To penetrate, he's going to push his penis downward with his fingers at the base of it, and slowly enter her. This can be quite stressful for a man's penis, so it's important to be extra lubed up and go very slowly.

WARNING: If this move hurts *at all*, stop immediately! Remember to thrust slowly. In rare cases, a penis can fracture when enough pressure is put on it.

WHERE TO DO IT The Missionary Reversed sex position is best performed on a wide open space like the bed. Because you need to be focused on doing this correctly, you don't want to be crammed in the car or even on the sofa for this one.

PROPS YOU'LL NEED Make sure to use lots of lube! You'll both need to be good and slick before attempting this position.

DIFFICULTY LEVEL ★★★★★

HER O-METER ★★★★★ She'll dig this sex position because the man has to do the gymnastics on this one!

HIS O-METER ★★★★★ It's going to take a very brave man to be able to do this sex position and get off on it.

> **MAKE IT HOTTER . . .** Use a liberator wedge to make the angle of penetration better for most men.

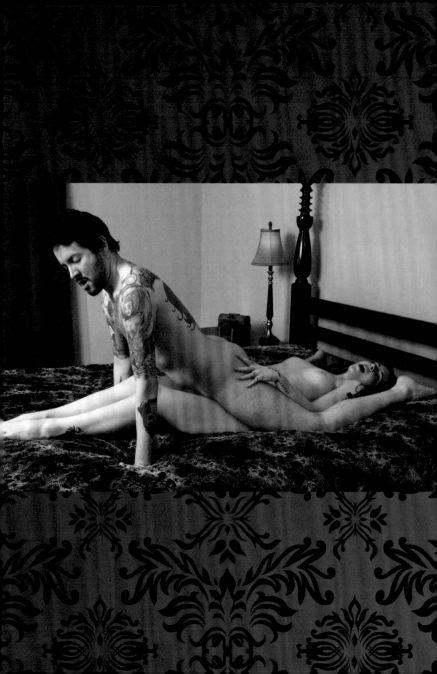

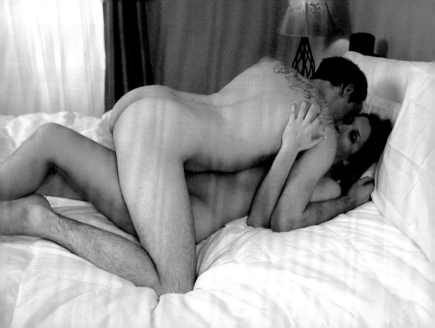

reverse jockey

The Reverse Jockey sex position is a fun twist on the traditional Missionary that allows him to be in complete control of the thrusting and stimulation. In this position, he sits atop his partner much like a jockey sits atop a racing horse, leaning forward and downward with the movement.

HOW TO DO IT The female partner lies on her back à la the traditional Missionary position. The male partner "mounts" his lady facing her head, but instead of putting his legs in between her slightly spread legs, he'll place them on either side of her. When he thrusts, he's going to lean forward and down and move his entire body instead of just his hips and buttocks.

WHERE TO DO IT This is a great sex position to use anywhere there is a narrow space and neither partner can spread their legs wide. The bed, sofa, and back seat of the car are all great options.

PROPS YOU'LL NEED None.

DIFFICULTY LEVEL ★★★★★

HER O-METER ☆☆☆★★ The Reverse Jockey sex position is good for her because there is more friction between her and her partner when her legs are pressed together. This is a good position for clitoral stimulation.

HIS O-METER ☆☆☆☆★ With her legs pressed together, her vagina feels much tighter to him. Although he won't be able to penetrate as deeply here as with other sex positions, the Reverse Jockey sex position will squeeze his penis firmly, creating an entirely new sensation for him.

MAKE IT HOTTER . . . The Reverse Jockey sex position is an excellent "male dominant" sex position. Take this a step further by incorporating a little BDSM (see chapter 10) or role play where she is in the submissive role.

x marks the spot

X Marks the Spot is a fun sex position that can be done on the bed or a table.

HOW TO DO IT In X Marks the Spot, the woman lies on the bed or table with her legs elevated and ankles crossed. The male partner enters her by holding on to her legs or crossed ankles. It's a fairly simple sex position to get into but is lots of fun for both partners! X Marks the Spot can be used for traditional rear entry vaginal sex, or it can be used for anal sex as well.

WHERE TO DO IT The kitchen table, dining room table, desk in the home office, and, of course, the bed would work for this sex position.

PROPS YOU'LL NEED Putting a towel down first and propping her head up on a pillow may make the hard surface more comfortable for her.

DIFFICULTY LEVEL ★★☆☆☆

HER O-METER ★★★☆☆ The deeper penetration is good for g-spot stimulation. The only thing that would make this sex position better is if he could grind against her clitoris. Unfortunately, he can't because her legs are crossed.

HIS O-METER ★★★☆☆ He likes X Marks the Spot because it's easy on him too. He simply gets to stand and thrust! Her crossed legs make for a tight vaginal entrance that feels divine, but he doesn't get to see a whole lot here with her legs in the way.

> **MAKE IT HOTTER . . .** A hands-free clitoral vibrator (one that can be worn) is a great option for X Marks the Spot if she needs more clitoral stimulation.

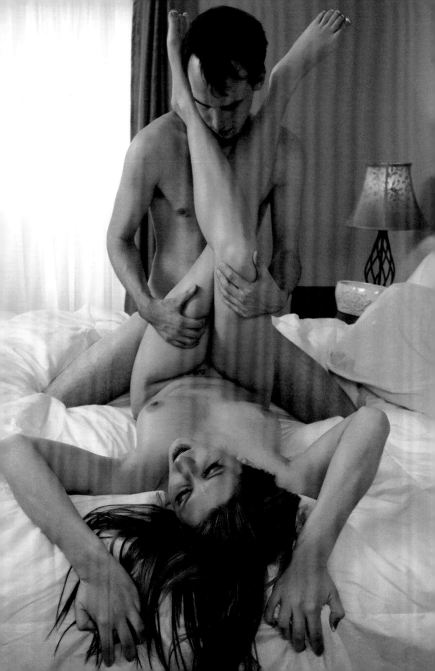

chapter 2: woman on top sex positions

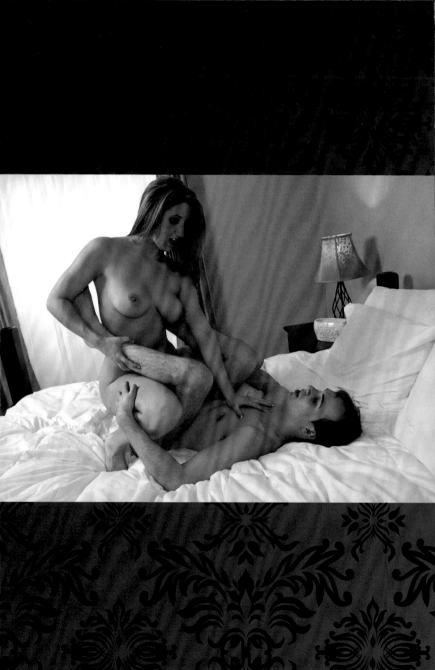

amazon

The Amazon sex position is an exotic form of woman-on-top that's easy for her, and it's great if he wants to be submissive.

HOW TO DO IT The male partner lies on his back and raises his legs, bringing his knees up to his chest with his legs parted. The female partner then straddles his groin with his knees in front of her and his legs wrapped around her waist, with his feet at her back. The Amazon sex position puts the female partner in total control of the thrusting, but it can be a bit difficult due to the angle at which his penis must bend to enter her.

WARNING: If this is at all uncomfortable or painful for the male partner, stop immediately!

WHERE TO DO IT The bed, floor, sofa, or backseat of the car are all fine for this position.

PROPS YOU'LL NEED Place a pillow under his head for comfort.

DIFFICULTY LEVEL ★★★★★

HER O-METER ★★★☆☆ The dominant woman will enjoy the control over thrusting that this position affords. G-spot orgasms can be had in the Amazon sex position, but she must be careful not to ride him too hard or put too much stress on his penis since it is bent at such an odd angle.

HIS O-METER ★☆☆☆☆ He can get off in this sex position, but it may not be easy for him. A super submissive man may really enjoy being dominated in this way, with his legs in the air and his buttocks exposed.

MAKE IT HOTTER . . . If he enjoys prostate massage, she can reach around and play with his anus during lovemaking for an explosive orgasm. If she can't reach around very well, a small butt plug or string of anal beads might be another option.

---

cowgirl

The Cowgirl is by far the most conducive to female orgasms, and many women can only orgasm in this position. Guys love it too because they get to sit back and relax while their girls take care of most of the thrusting action. This is a must-have sex position in your repertoire.

HOW TO DO IT The Cowgirl is a favorite among women! It's also known as the "Woman on Top" sex position. The male partner lies flat on his back (like the woman does in standard Missionary) and the female partner straddles his pelvis with her legs on either side of him, resting her weight on her knees. He can bend his knees some to help support her, or he can leave his legs lying flat on the bed. She can sit straight up, but it is more common for women to lean forward some for more clitoral stimulation.

WHERE TO DO IT The sofa, bed, chair, floor, or car—any flat surface will do for the Cowgirl.

PROPS YOU'LL NEED A soft blanket or pillow to go under her knees will really help!

DIFFICULTY LEVEL ★★★★

HER O-METER ★★★★★ The Cowgirl allows a woman to control almost everything about sex—the speed and depth of penetration as well as the angle. She can change any one of these things to better facilitate an orgasm, and this makes it much easier for her to achieve the big O. Because this sex position offers such excellent g-spot and clitoral stimulation, many women can have blended orgasms!

HIS O-METER ★★★★★ If she's getting off, he's getting off. He really loves watching her do her thing, so this sex position gives him a great show. He really digs her riding him and using his body to get herself off.

MAKE IT HOTTER . . . If she's sitting straight up, he's got a much better view, and she can touch herself while having sex to give him the ultimate show!

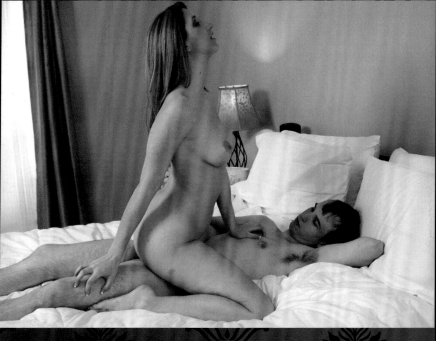

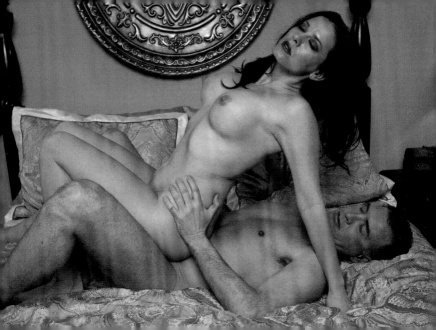

hot seat

The Hot Seat sex position is a combination between woman on top and rear entry. It's perfect for when you're craving something a little naughty but not too difficult.

HOW TO DO IT The male partner lies down with his legs spread, knees bent, and feet flat on the bed or floor. The female partner lowers herself onto her lover facing away from him, with her back to him and her legs bent in a similar way to his. Her hands are on the bed or floor beside his torso to allow her to bear her own weight and use her muscles for thrusting and rocking her pelvis back and forth. You may only be able to achieve a grinding or rocking movement in this position, but many couples will enjoy how slow and sensual it is.

WHERE TO DO IT The Hot Seat is great for the sofa or a sturdy reclining chair, although it can also be done on the bed with pillows under the male partner for support.

PROPS YOU'LL NEED He'll appreciate lots of pillows to lounge on while enjoying the show.

DIFFICULTY LEVEL ★★★★★

HER O-METER ★★★★★ Her arms can get plenty tired in the Hot Seat, and there's little clitoral action going on here. However, the angle of penetration is such that it affords excellent g-spot stimulation! She may be able to coax herself to orgasm here, especially if she reaches down and stimulates her clitoris with her hand or a sex toy.

HIS O-METER ★★★★★ Do this one in front of a mirror so that he can watch the show. It will make the Hot Seat much sexier for him.

> **MAKE IT HOTTER . . .** If the female partner has enough upper arm strength to lift herself up and down during lovemaking, it will allow her partner to see himself sliding in and out of her, greatly increasing how hot the Hot Seat is for him!

crab

The Crab is a unique woman-on-top sex position that gives the male partner quite a show during lovemaking, even if it is awkward for him to do.

HOW TO DO IT The male partner lies on his back with his legs spread a little, and the female partner sits on top of him, with her feet facing him. She can lean back and grab on to his feet to help with thrusting, or she can use her legs, which are bent so that her feet rest flat on the floor or bed on either side of her partner's torso. Although the Crab allows the male partner to view penetration, it can be a difficult sex position for him to master because his penis is bent at an odd angle. It's not impossible though, and men who have flexible penises will likely enjoy this sex position.

WARNING: Any discomfort or pain means stop immediately! Play it safe and find another sex position if you find this one hurts.

WHERE TO DO IT The Crab can be done on any flat surface, but you'll both probably appreciate the comfort of a bed.

PROPS YOU'LL NEED He may want a pillow or two under his head to help support him so he can see the action if he's not propped up on his elbows.

DIFFICULTY LEVEL ★★★★★

HER O-METER ★★★☆☆ While the Crab doesn't afford her much clitoral stimulation on its own, her partner can easily reach for her clitoris and stimulate it during thrusting with his hands (which will make the show even more fun!). She may really enjoy the dominance of this sex position, even if getting the hang of thrusting is a little challenging.

HIS O-METER ★★★☆☆ If he can get into the Crab comfortably, it's likely to be an exceptionally enjoyable position for him because he can see everything that is going on. However, if it is uncomfortable or his penis isn't flexible, he's not likely to enjoy as well, if at all. Go slow until you get the hang of how to thrust and move in this sex position.

MAKE IT HOTTER . . . He can stimulate her clitoris and labia, or he can use a sex toy on her. Both of these things make the Crab even hotter than it already is!

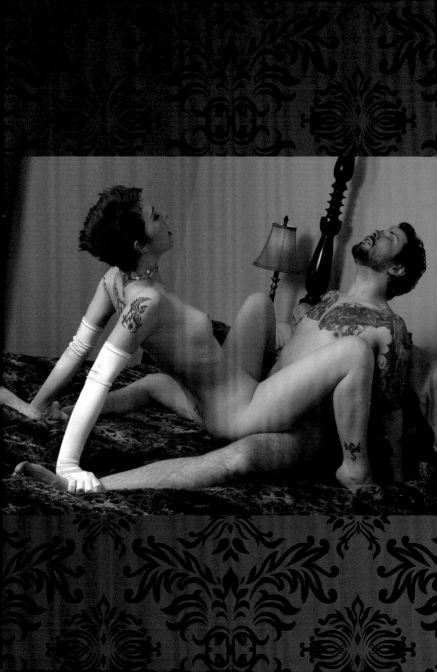

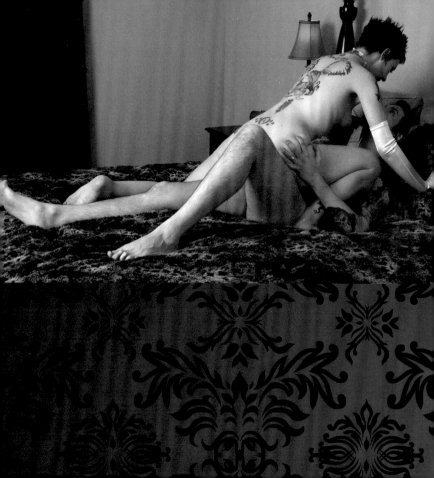

The Lunge is a fun twist on woman on top that allows for super deep penetration. The only trick is that the female partner must be quite flexible.

HOW TO DO IT The male partner lies on his back on the bed. The female partner straddles him (almost as though this was Cowgirl but with her playing the role of the man) and raises one leg up and hooks it around his hip, resting her foot on the bed and against the outside of his buttocks. The other leg is straight back and flush with the bed. The Lunge gets its name because it looks like the female is doing a "lunge" type of stretch as she lowers herself onto his penis.

WHERE TO DO IT This is one you'll want to do on a bed. You'll want all the comfort and space you can get here.

PROPS YOU'LL NEED A pillow for him is nice, especially if he wants his head supported so he can see more of the action.

DIFFICULTY LEVEL ★★★★★

HER O-METER ★★★★★ Although the Lunge allows for fairly good clitoral friction and excellent deep penetration and g-spot stimulation, it can be quite difficult for a woman to get into and stay in—and even harder for her to figure out how to thrust in. She must be pretty flexible to pull this off comfortably, but if she can, the mix between clitoral friction and deep g-spot stimulation can result in some powerful orgasms.

HIS O-METER ★★★★★ He likes the Lunge because it allows him to lie back, relax, and enjoy her taking control. He also likes to watch her here, because if she lifts the bent leg ever so slightly, it provides him with a pretty decent view of the action.

MAKE IT HOTTER . . . He can reach up and play with her nipples in the Lunge, or if both partners are feeling extra naughty, he can reach around to her backside for some anal play, since the position of her legs leaves her anal area exposed.

rearview mirror

If you're looking for an exotic yet easy rear entry sex position, the Rearview Mirror will definitely fit the bill. It's fun to try!

HOW TO DO IT The male partner sits on a surface like the floor or bed with his legs stretched out, and spread apart slightly so his lover can fit in between them. The female partner then lies on her stomach in between his legs with her head facing his feet, and her legs spread wide enough to allow his torso in between them. It may take some practice to align your groins perfectly, but it is possible!

In this position, he won't be able to do much of the thrusting, so she will be in charge of the rhythm and depth of the thrusts. The Rearview Mirror is similar to the Reverse Cowgirl (see page 49) so if this one feels awkward, try that one first.

WHERE TO DO IT Since a fair amount of space is required for this position, you'll want to do it on the floor or the bed. A sofa or another narrow space just isn't going to work out as well.

PROPS YOU'LL NEED A blanket or thick towel will make this position more comfortable on the floor.

DIFFICULTY LEVEL ★★★★★

HER O-METER ★★★★★ While the Rearview Mirror is fairly comfortable for her, the angle of penetration may be a bit awkward at first, as well as getting the hang of thrusting. In this sex position, it's less actual "thrusting," and more of a rocking, grinding motion. This, however, can help stimulate her clitoris for more orgasm potential!

HIS O-METER ★★★★★ He likes the view in the Rearview Mirror; however, it may be a bit of an awkward angle for his penis to bend.

WARNING: If there is any discomfort in this sex position, stop immediately!

MAKE IT HOTTER . . . His hands are in the perfect position to spank her bottom or even engage in some anal play if she's okay with it. That can make the Rearview Mirror position even naughtier!

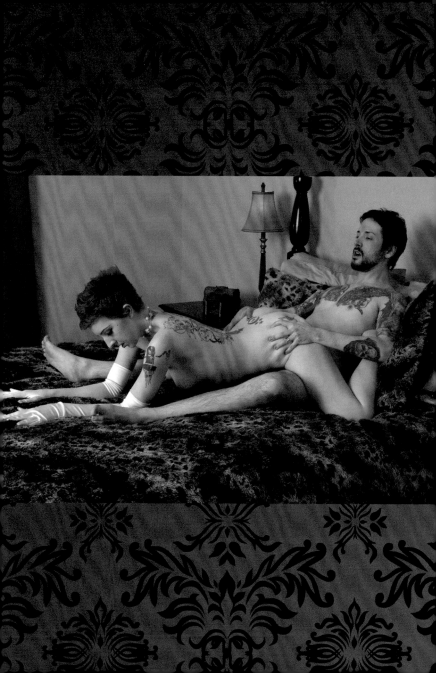

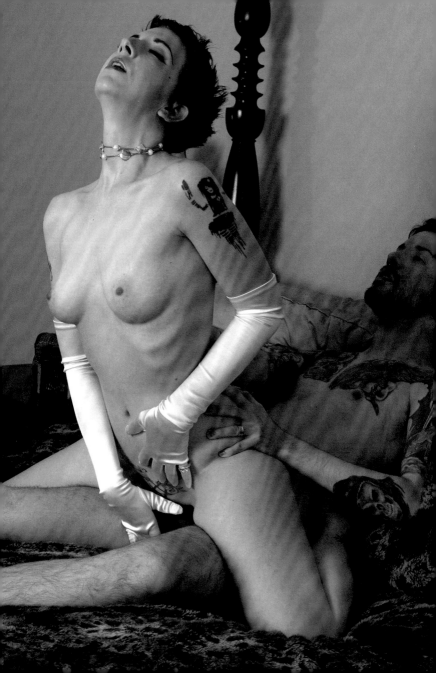

reverse cowgirl

The Reverse Cowgirl is one of the best sex positions for a guy, because he gets quite the view while she rides him up and down. It's not quite as orgasmic as the Cowgirl is for a woman, but it's a little kinkier and can be a lot of fun for both partners.

HOW TO DO IT Instead of straddling her lover facing him, the female partner straddles him facing his feet, again with one leg on either side of him with her weight resting on her knees.

WHERE TO DO IT Try this one on the bed, sofa, floor, or back seat of the car—anywhere you have space to lie down!

PROPS YOU'LL NEED None.

DIFFICULTY LEVEL ★☆☆☆☆

HER O-METER ★★★☆☆ The Reverse Cowgirl isn't as powerful for a woman as the Cowgirl is. While she still gets to control the speed, depth, and angle of penetration, because she's facing her lover's feet, his anatomy doesn't line up to her hot spots as well. It's still possible for her to get g-spot stimulation from his penis, but not as easily because the penis is rubbing the wall of her vagina that her g-spot isn't on.

HIS O-METER ★★★★★ Men really love the Reverse Cowgirl. It gives them as much visual stimulation as many rear entry sex positions do, but it combines the excitement of her controlling the action. If a woman wants to surprise her man with a super-hot sex position, the Reverse Cowgirl is the way to go.

> **MAKE IT HOTTER . . .** Ladies, lean forward quite a bit and let your rear take center stage here. Give yourself a good trim or shave, and make sure you're clean and smelling nice.

The Seated Scissors sex position is a fun way for her to be on top and get great clitoral stimulation too.

HOW TO DO IT The male partner lies on his back on a bed and spreads his legs with one knee bent. His partner gets on top of him and intertwines her legs with his. She is facing away from him and straddling his thigh so that her groin is pressed against his leg and he is able to penetrate her. It's similar to Reverse Cowgirl, but she is riding his leg instead of his torso.

WHERE TO DO IT The Seated Scissors sex position requires so much space that you're better off doing it on the bed. While the floor will work, the bed is certainly the most comfortable option. If you do decide to do it on the floor, make sure you have plenty of blankets and pillows! It's also a fun sex position to do outdoors on a picnic blanket if you have enough privacy!

PROPS YOU'LL NEED Blankets and pillows, depending on where you are.

DIFFICULTY LEVEL ★★★★★

HER O-METER ★★★★★ She likes the Seated Scissors sex position because it's exceptionally easy for her to get clitoral stimulation. She can grind her clitoris up against his thigh, and with some lube, it can feel absolutely fantastic. And unlike traditional Scissors (see page 144), she is in full control of the movement.

HIS O-METER ★★★★★ He likes watching her enjoy this one! Because she is in control, it may not be as orgasmic for him as some of the other positions.

MAKE IT HOTTER . . . Increase his orgasmic potential by performing this position in front of a mirror so that he can get a great view of her backside and her facial expressions as she pleasures herself.

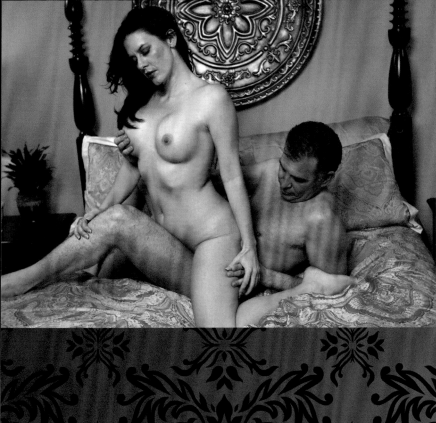

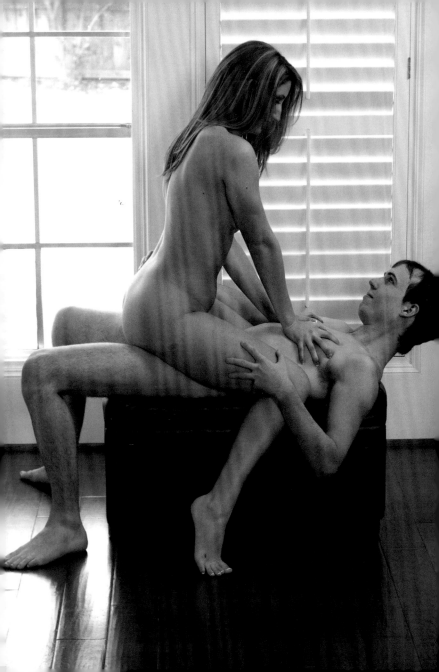

sybian

Just like Sybian sex toys, the Sybian sex position allows the female partner to be in complete control and thrust and grind herself to orgasm.

HOW TO DO IT The male partner lies back on an ottoman or small table, with his feet flat on the floor. The chosen piece of furniture should be long enough so that his head and hips are supported, and only his feet and legs are draped over the side. The female partner straddles his hips and lowers herself onto his penis while facing him, and uses him to grind and thrust her way to a g-spot or clitoral orgasm—or both!

WHERE TO DO IT This one is best performed on a large ottoman or long, narrow coffee table.

PROPS YOU'LL NEED Other than the right size furniture, you really don't need anything extra for this one.

DIFFICULTY LEVEL ★★★☆☆

HER O-METER ★★★★☆ Since she is in complete control here, she can give herself as much or as little clitoral friction as she needs to orgasm. She can also choose what depth and speed to thrust at, stimulating her g-spot in just the right way. The Sybian sex position is named after the popular Sybian sex toy, which is a mountable toy that allows a woman to ride herself to complete bliss. Doing it with a real person can be just as satisfying, if not more so!

HIS O-METER ★★★★☆ He enjoys laying back and allowing his partner to be in control every once in a while, and for guys who don't know much about how to give a woman an orgasm during intercourse, the Sybian sex position is an excellent option since she takes the reins and is responsible for giving herself an orgasm while using his "equipment." He also enjoys the view!

> **MAKE IT HOTTER . . .** He is your toy in this position so enjoy the ride and give him a good show!

side saddle

The Side Saddle sex position is a unique twist on woman on top and can be fun for both partners, but it is a little more difficult for her than it is him.

HOW TO DO IT The male partner lies on the edge of the bed or the sofa, completely flat. The female partner stands at his hips, facing away from him, and lowers herself onto his groin, with her feet still on the floor. Her body will be perpendicular to his, and she will be facing away from him throughout lovemaking. She will use her legs and arms to push herself up and down on his penis.

WHERE TO DO IT The Side Saddle is best performed on the sofa or the edge of the bed, but a lounge chair by the pool may be fun as well.

PROPS YOU'LL NEED He may want a pillow, but it's not essential, especially if you're on a comfortable surface like the sofa or bed.

DIFFICULTY LEVEL ★★★☆☆

HER O-METER ★☆☆☆☆ This can be a difficult sex position for her to master and enjoy, simply because she is responsible for all the movement during sex. The Side Saddle sex position requires substantial strength in the arms and legs, and a certain amount of stamina and endurance as well. If your leg and arm muscles aren't used to physical strain, you might feel them start to burn after just a few minutes of moving yourself up and down. However, athletic women may truly enjoy the control they have in this sex position!

HIS O-METER ★★★☆ The Side Saddle sex position is a breeze for him, because all he's doing is laying there! He's quite comfortable here and can relax and enjoy the sensations as long as his lover can keep it up. He'll enjoy letting her "take the reins" for a little while!

MAKE IT HOTTER . . . She can make the Side Saddle sex position more enjoyable if she thinks of her man as a "living Sybian sex toy." He is a penis for her to ride and enjoy. He, by the way, will greatly enjoy her confidence and freedom!

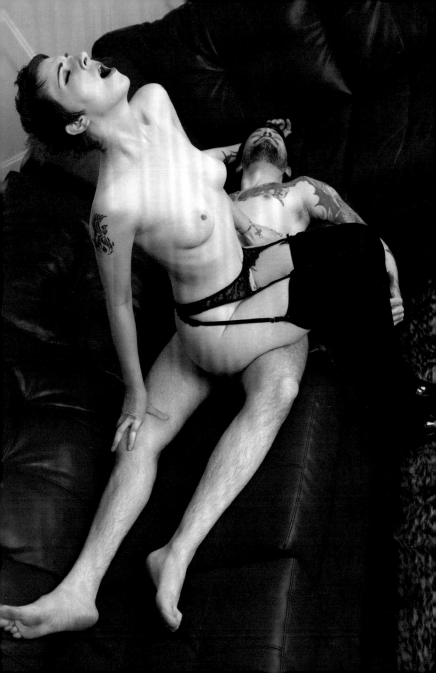

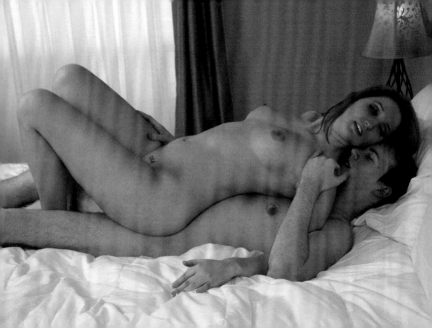

sunny side up

The Sunny Side Up sex position is an interesting twist on both rear entry and woman on top. She'll love this sex position as much as he does!

HOW TO DO IT The male partner lies on a flat surface face up, and his partner lies on top of him, also face up so her back is pressed against his torso. He enters her this way from behind and grasps her hips to help push her up and down on top of him. This is both a somewhat exotic yet sweet and sensual sex position that both partners will enjoy! However, this is not a good sex position to try if the female partner is on the heavy side because it will be much more difficult for him to stay comfortable and lift her hips up and down.

WHERE TO DO IT The Sunny Side Up is an excellent sex position for the backseat of the car or the sofa if you're looking for something other than your traditional Missionary to try in these places.

PROPS YOU'LL NEED He will be very grateful for a pillow under his head!

DIFFICULTY LEVEL ★★★★★

HER O-METER ★★★★★ She loves the intimacy of the Sunny Side Up sex position and enjoys it fairly well, but it's not particularly orgasmic for her unless her lover reaches around and stimulates her clitoris, or she does it herself.

HIS O-METER ★★★★★ His arms may tire some from lifting his partner's hips up and down to facilitate thrusting, but he will enjoy the closeness and uniqueness that the Sunny Side Up sex position has to offer. It's definitely on his "must try" list! He'll really enjoy reaching up and fondling her breasts as she grinds against him.

MAKE IT HOTTER . . . This is a great sex position for the adventurous couple who enjoys anal sex, because it provides a more intimate way to engage in anal than traditional anal sex positions like Doggy Style. She can make the Sunny Side Up sex position super hot by using a clitoral vibrator on herself while she grinds against her lover's groin!

chapter 3: oral sex positions for her

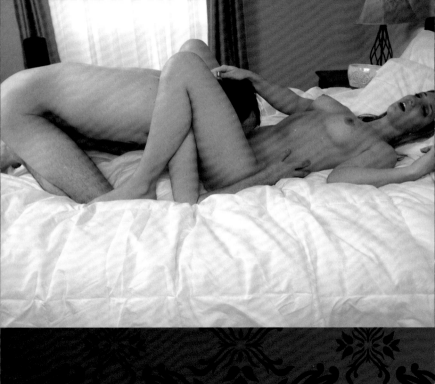

spread eagle

This classic oral sex position is a tried and true standard for many couples. Although it lacks the "exotic" factor, it's a favorite among women because they can simply lie back, relax, and enjoy the pleasure!

HOW TO DO IT This is the "Missionary" of oral sex positions for her. It's the most common oral sex position for women, and it's actually a favorite, simply because the female partner has the ability to relax and focus on the pleasurable sensations she's receiving. For many women, relaxation and focus are critical components to achieving orgasm! The female partner lies on her back with her legs spread, and her male partner situates himself in between her legs so that he can give her oral sex. It's simple, but very, very effective!

WHERE TO DO IT While this position can be done just about anywhere, the comfort of a soft bed will help her relax and enjoy herself more.

PROPS YOU'LL NEED Adding a pillow under her lower back will tilt her pelvis up and give her partner more access to her vulva.

DIFFICULTY LEVEL ★☆☆☆☆

HER O-METER ★★★★★ Women love the Spread Eagle because they're able to lie back, relax, and enjoy everything. They only have to focus on what feels good, which can be exactly what a woman needs to reach orgasm.

HIS O-METER ★☆☆☆☆ This is probably the least favorite oral sex position among men, simply because it can make for some serious neck cramps! It's not easy getting the angle right when licking, and the neck can bend in an odd way. Some men may not be able to keep this position up long enough to actually bring their lovers to orgasm. He also can't reach down and stimulate himself very well.

> **MAKE IT HOTTER . . .** Guys, slip a lubed finger inside her vagina and gently massage her g-spot while you lick her clitoris (after she's warmed up and turned on, of course!) This will increase her chances of orgasm, and if you do it well enough, you may even get her to squirt!

bottoms up

The Bottoms Up is an oral sex position that puts her in an extremely vulnerable, yet naughty and erotic pose! It's only for the adventurous!

HOW TO DO IT The female partner lies on her back, grasps her hips and raises her buttocks in the air, letting her legs fall back towards her head. The male partner rests his weight on his knees and helps hold her hips for stability as he goes down on her from above. What makes the Bottoms Up so incredibly naughty is that it completely exposes both her vulva and anal areas for him to stimulate with his mouth as he pleases. This is an oral sex position that should definitely only be performed by couples who are extremely comfortable with each other.

WHERE TO DO IT The bed is the best place for the Bottoms Up.

PROPS YOU'LL NEED She may want a pillow for her neck and upper shoulders. A Liberator Wedge is a great way for her to easily stay in position without getting too tired from holding herself up.

DIFFICULTY LEVEL ★★★★★

HER O-METER ★★★★☆ If she's super adventurous and kinky, she will absolutely love the Bottoms Up. She'll love feeling spread out and vulnerable to her partner! If she's not very flexible, however, this position may be fairly uncomfortable for her.

HIS O-METER ★★★★☆ He will enjoy the Bottoms Up if he really digs giving oral sex, or even if he likes giving analingus. This sex position doesn't force him to crane his neck in any way, making it one of the more comfortable oral sex positions for him.

MAKE IT HOTTER . . . If he doesn't want to perform analingus but still wants to introduce anal play to make the Bottoms Up even kinkier, he can use his fingers or a small anal toy to stimulate that area while he licks and sucks on her clitoris.

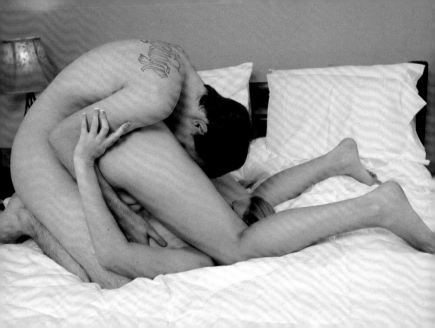

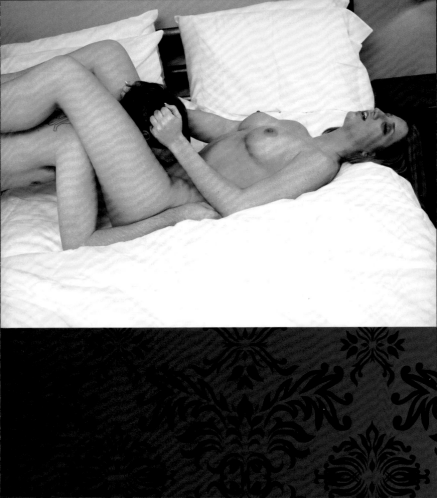

ear warmer

The Ear Warmer sex position is a simple variation of the Spread Eagle (see page 61), where she has more control and may be more comfortable than with her legs spread.

HOW TO DO IT The female partner lies back and spreads her legs long enough for her partner to lie on his stomach and place his head in between to give her oral sex. Instead of keeping her legs spread like with the Spread Eagle sex position, she closes her legs somewhat, resting her inner thighs on either side of her lover's head. This gives her more control during cunnilingus, and many women may be more comfortable with their hips at this angle.

WHERE TO DO IT The bed is a super comfortable and familiar area to perform this position, but it can also be done on the edge of the bed (with her partner resting his knees on the floor) or on a sofa.

PROPS YOU'LL NEED Add a pillow for her head and possibly under her lower back to place her hips at an angle that makes oral sex easier for him to give.

DIFFICULTY LEVEL ★★★★

HER O-METER ★★★★★ With increased control and comfort, she can really lie back and relax in the Ear Warmer sex position. She loves receiving oral sex, and in this position he's totally and completely focusing on her pleasure.

HIS O-METER ★★★★★ The Ear Warmer sex position may not be his favorite if he wants to have more freedom for head movement. He may feel a little confined with her legs pressed up against his head.

MAKE IT HOTTER . . . He can easily use one of his hands to stimulate her g-spot while he's licking her clitoris, which will bring her to orgasm even faster.

face straddle

The Face Straddle is an excellent oral sex position to use when the female partner wants to feel in control of oral sex, and the male partner wants to feel a little submissive. It also gives him a great view of her body as she writhes in pleasure!

HOW TO DO IT The male partner assumes a lying position and the female partner lowers her genitals over his face, straddling his head with each leg on one side of his head. There are a couple of ways to do this, but both require her to rest her weight on her knees. She can lean back and rest the remainder of her weight on her hands, or she can lean forward and get on all fours. Either way, this provides her lover with complete access to her genitals.

WHERE TO DO IT Try the sofa, bed, floor, or back seat of the car—anywhere with enough space to lie down.

PROPS YOU'LL NEED A pillow for his neck is a definite must!

DIFFICULTY LEVEL ★☆☆☆☆

HER O-METER ★★★★☆ This is an excellent oral sex position for her because she feels more in control here. She can move her pelvis to guide her clitoris to where she wants it to be, and she can rock and move in a way that gets her closer to orgasm. She's not relying only on him to get her there.

HIS O-METER ★★★☆☆ Many men enjoy this position, because they feel a little submissive here. Also, if a man isn't that confident at oral sex, he may feel better that she can maneuver herself so that she gets more pleasure, rather than relying only on him and his tongue movements to get her off.

MAKE IT HOTTER . . . Guys, reach down and masturbate while you're giving her oral sex. She won't necessarily be able to look behind her to see what you're doing, but the idea that you love eating her out so much that you can't help but touch yourself is extremely erotic for her, especially considering that many women feel that guys think oral sex is a chore.

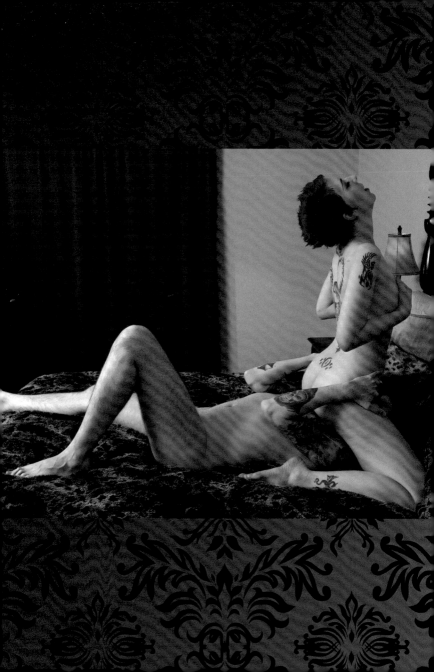

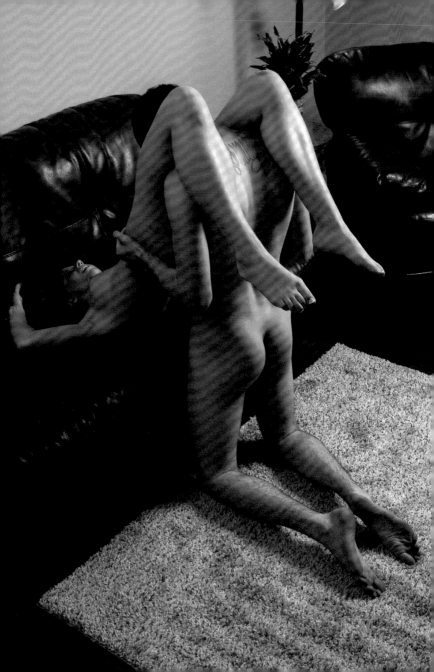

feedbag

The Feedbag is an interesting oral sex position that can be a little challenging for her but is very rewarding once it is accomplished.

HOW TO DO IT The female partner lies on the sofa with her rear at the edge of it and her legs and feet hanging off. Her partner then kneels in front of her, lifts her buttocks with his hands and places her legs over his shoulders. It's a tight fit for his head to get in between her legs, but it can be a lot of fun once he's there.

WHERE TO DO IT The sofa is the best place for the Feedbag.

PROPS YOU'LL NEED She may want a small pillow for her neck and upper shoulders, and he'll appreciate a pillow, blanket, or towel for his knees to rest on instead of the floor.

DIFFICULTY LEVEL ★★★★★

HER O-METER ★★★★★ The Feedbag probably isn't going to be her favorite position for oral sex, but hey, she's getting it, so it's all good, right? Her legs aren't spread very wide at all here, so her lover has limited access to the nerves on her inner labia and even parts of her clitoris. She's also in a bit of an awkward position; however, the blood rushing to her head can intensify her orgasm if he can get her there.

HIS O-METER ★★★★★ If he really likes being enveloped by his lover's vulva and legs, he's going to love the Feedbag, but he'll likely enjoy other oral sex positions if he wants more control or freedom of movement.

MAKE IT HOTTER . . . He can easily reach forward and caress her thighs and belly, as well as stimulating her breasts and nipples with his hands!

leg up

This hot oral sex position for her is simple for both partners. The Leg Up gives him full access to her, while making it easy for her to watch.

HOW TO DO IT The female partner stands next to a chair, sofa, low table, or other surface and raises one leg at a ninety-degree angle so she can rest her foot on the surface and spread her legs. Her partner sits on the floor cross-legged beneath her, with his head positioned in between her legs. He can grasp her hips or play with her breasts while he goes down on her in the Leg Up sex position.

WHERE TO DO IT You can do the Leg Up anywhere you can put one foot up!

PROPS YOU'LL NEED A chair, sofa, low table, or bed that is the proper height for her to rest her foot on so that she is comfortable. He may also want a pillow, small blanket, or towel to sit on, as he will be sitting on the floor.

DIFFICULTY LEVEL ★ ☆ ☆ ☆ ☆

HER O-METER ★ ★ ★ ☆ What she loves about the Leg Up is that she's not only comfortable but spread open wide enough for him to access her most sensitive parts. She can watch the action here, which is not always the case in other oral sex positions. This is an entirely new way for her to experience oral sex! The one downside is that it may be difficult to reach orgasm from the standing position.

HIS O-METER ★ ★ ★ ★ ★ He's comfortable in the Leg Up too, and loves being able to grasp her buttocks or raise his hands up and fondle her breasts while he goes down on her.

MAKE IT HOTTER . . . Her hands are fairly unoccupied in the Leg Up, so she can use them to either stimulate her own nipples or reach down and spread her labia wide for him. The latter will take the Leg Up up a few notches and make it way hotter than it already is!

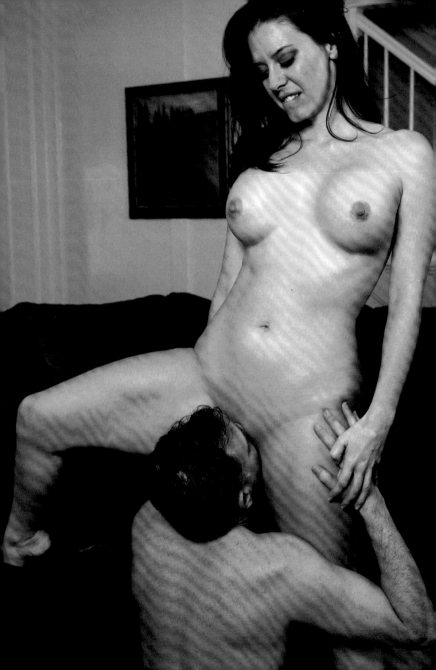

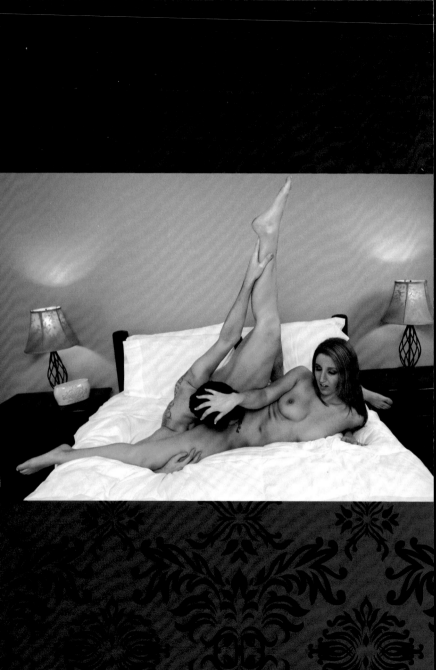

licking the flagpole

Licking the Flagpole is a comfortable oral sex position for both her and him, which leaves her spread wide open for the ultimate pleasure.

HOW TO DO IT Licking the Flagpole is easy to get into. The female partner simply lies on her side on the bed, with her bottom leg bent at the knee to give her stability. She then lifts her top leg high in the air, placing her hand on her thigh to help hold it up. The male partner then lies on his side perpendicular to her and rests his head on her bottom thigh while he goes down on her.

WHERE TO DO IT This is okay on a floor or other wide open space, but both partners will appreciate the comfort of the bed with surrounding pillows.

PROPS YOU'LL NEED Use pillows as needed for extra support.

DIFFICULTY LEVEL ★☆☆☆☆

HER O-METER ★★★★☆ She loves being spread out for him, because this position gives him access to every nerve in her clitoris and labia. The only caveat is that if she's not very flexible or athletic, she may have trouble stretching her leg that high and keeping it there for a significant period of time. It's fine to put a slight bend in the knee of the top leg to make it more comfortable.

HIS O-METER ★★★☆☆ He enjoys the comfort of this position, and it's very easy on the neck. Since her inner thigh is supporting his head, he's quite comfortable and relaxed while giving her oral sex.

MAKE IT HOTTER . . . If she enjoys anal play, Licking the Flagpole is perfect for him to give her simultaneous oral sex and anal stimulation with his hands. It's a great way to make this sex position even naughtier than it already is!

One of the more "kinky" oral sex positions for her, the Reverse Face Straddle is not for the shy or timid woman. Because it involves her partner's face and nose so close to her backdoor, she needs to be super comfortable with her partner. But it's an excellent position for couples who enjoy anal play!

HOW TO DO IT As with the forward facing version of this oral sex position, the male partner lies on a bed, sofa, or the floor (any flat surface will do), and the female partner straddles his face, with one leg on either side of his head, resting her weight on her knees. The difference with this position is that she's facing his feet, as in the "Reverse Cowgirl" sex position. He is able to perform oral sex on her from behind, and this is actually an excellent oral sex position for couples who enjoy analingus. Because her rear is right in his face, she's clean and trimmed or shaved. He's going to feel better about it too!

WHERE TO DO IT The Reverse Straddle can be done on the sofa, back seat of the car, floor, or any flat surface.

PROPS YOU'LL NEED Use a pillow or rolled up towel to support the male partner's neck.

DIFFICULTY LEVEL ☆☆☆★★

HER O-METER ☆☆☆★★ This is an oral sex position that really kinky women enjoy!

HIS O-METER ☆☆☆★★ Men who like to be dominated (and men who like things a little kinky, or have a butt fetish) will really enjoy this oral sex position. Guys, you can up the pleasure factor for yourself by reaching down and masturbating while you're giving her oral sex. Since she's facing your feet, she'll be able to see you touch yourself and it will turn her on like you wouldn't believe!

MAKE IT HOTTER . . . If you're into analingus, this is the time to try it. Use a dental dam for ultimate safety. Definitely discuss this beforehand though. Guys, you don't want to surprise her with a tongue up her bum if she hasn't agreed to it first!

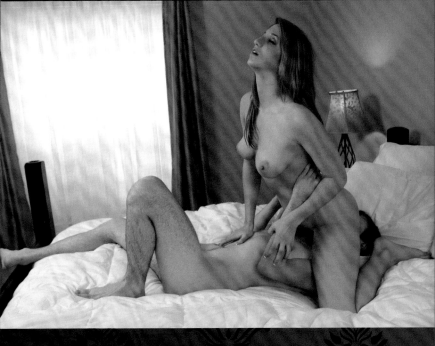

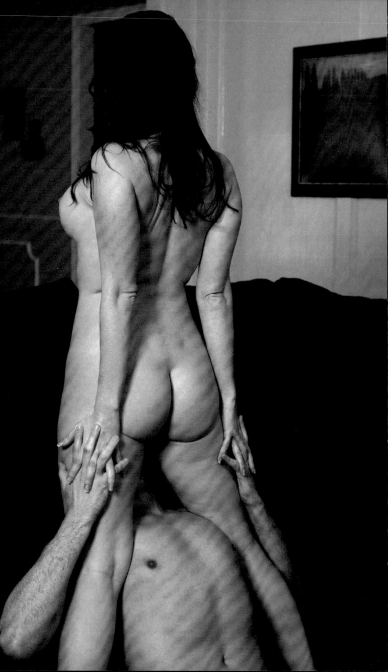

standing face straddle

The Standing Face Straddle is a fun and easy oral sex position that puts her in control. He likes it almost as much as she does!

HOW TO DO IT The male partner sits on the floor with his legs crossed, and his partner stands above him, lowering her groin onto his face. He holds onto her hips for more stability, and she can use her hands to caress her own breasts and stimulate her nipples. It's quick and easy, but it's a very satisfying oral sex position for her.

WHERE TO DO IT The Standing Face Straddle is awesome for an oral sex quickie, because it can be done pretty much anywhere you have enough space. He doesn't have to get undressed, and all she really has to do is drop her drawers!

PROPS YOU'LL NEED None.

DIFFICULTY LEVEL ★★★★★

HER O-METER ★★★★★ She loves being in control in the Standing Face Straddle, especially considering that she can easily grind against his face to achieve an intense orgasm.

HIS O-METER ★★★★★ Submissive guys will like the Standing Face Straddle; however, guys who like to be in control may not enjoy it as much. If she starts grinding too hard, it can become a bit uncomfortable. Communicate with your partner non-verbally if she starts to get a little too aggressive or you feel like you're suffocating!

MAKE IT HOTTER . . . He can use his fingers to stimulate her g-spot while she can control the tempo and depth of her thrusting. It's the best of both worlds. A good g-spot vibrator is an incredible addition to this position!

under the hood (for her)

The Under the Hood position is one that gives her partner full access to her nether region and makes her feel exceptionally exposed.

HOW TO DO IT The female partner lies on her back, and brings her legs and knees as close to her chest as possible. Typically, her legs are stretched out, but if this is difficult for her to do, a slight bend in the knee is okay. She can hold the backs of her thighs to help support her legs. The male partner then kneels to give his partner oral sex.

WHERE TO DO IT A wide space like the bed or floor is best for the Under the Hood, but the bed is of course going to be much more comfortable.

PROPS YOU'LL NEED She will want a pillow under her head, and he'll want one under his knees if he's on the floor. A rolled up blanket or towel will also work.

DIFFICULTY LEVEL ★☆☆☆☆

HER O-METER ★★★★☆ If she's not comfortable with her anal area being exposed, she's not going to like this sex position very much. However, for women who are totally comfortable with themselves, this one is a must try! It's totally hot!

HIS O-METER ★★★☆☆ He likes the Under the Hood position because it gives her the opportunity to feel vulnerable and him the opportunity to be in complete control.

MAKE IT HOTTER . . . For a bondage twist, restrain her hands with ties and hold her legs in the fully spread position while giving her pleasure.

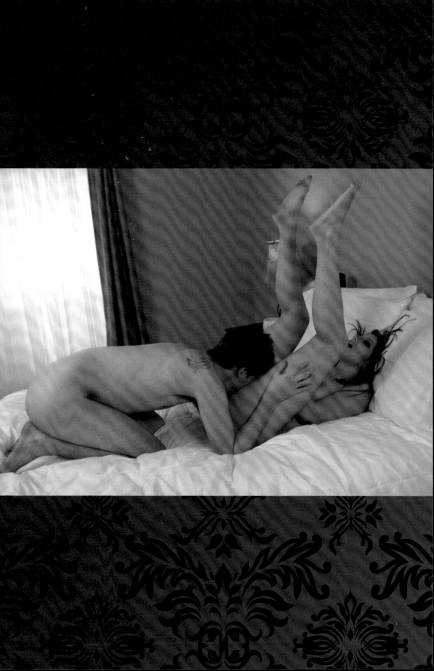

chapter 4: oral sex positions for him

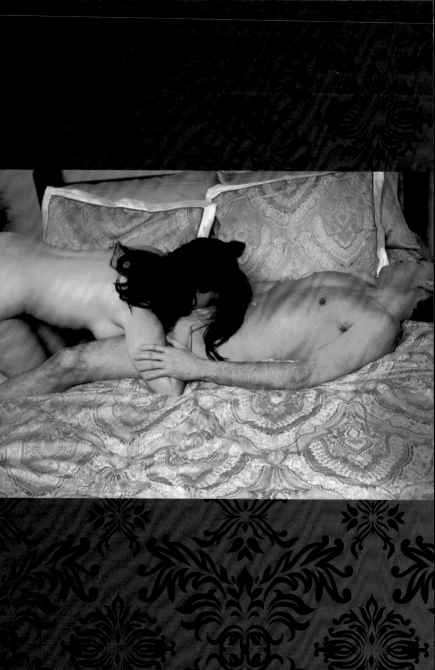

the original

The "chicken soup" of oral sex positions for him, the Original is probably one of his favorite ways to receive a blowjob. It allows him to lie back and relax while he receives pleasure, and it's not terribly difficult for her to do either.

HOW TO DO IT The male partner lies back, propped up against pillows or even flat on his back, while his partner kneels over him to give oral sex. His legs are spread enough so that she can get in between them, and she can either support her weight on her knees or lie flat on her stomach.

WHERE TO DO IT The Original can be done on the bed, sofa, floor, and perhaps even the car! This is a very versatile oral sex position for both partners. Feel free to do it anywhere you see an opportunity to lie down!

PROPS YOU'LL NEED He may like some pillows to support his upper torso so he can watch the action.

DIFFICULTY LEVEL ★☆☆☆☆

HER O-METER ★☆☆☆☆ She likes the Original because it's easy, and he enjoys it. This is probably the first oral sex position a woman learns to do!

HIS O-METER ★★★★★ He loves the Original simply because it's tried and true. It may be the first kind of blowjob he ever received, so, of course, there are probably fond memories! He's lying back and relaxing while getting a blowjob, and if he's propped up, he gets to watch. It's simple, yet very, very effective.

MAKE IT HOTTER . . . Try playing with some submissive roles for her. A sex game where she's "serving" him can be a lot of fun when you incorporate the Original in the mix! Or, you can simply revel in the comfort that this oldie but goodie gives both partners.

---

almost 69

In the Almost 69, he's receiving a blowjob in the same position as 69, but without having to reciprocate. Very hot!

HOW TO DO IT Both partners lie on their sides as though they were about to assume the side-by-side 69 sex position, with each partner facing the other's feet. The female partner will proceed to give him oral sex, and while he is in the position to do the same for her, he doesn't. He simply relaxes and enjoys what she's doing to him!

WHERE TO DO IT The Almost 69 oral sex position can be done in a variety of places, especially narrow ones like the backseat of a car. Since both partners are lying side by side, not as much space is required. Use your imagination here!

PROPS YOU'LL NEED None.

DIFFICULTY LEVEL ★★★★

HER O-METER ★★★★ The Almost 69 oral sex position is comfortable for her, but she might just wish he would go down on her at the same time and turn it into a regular 69!

HIS O-METER ★★★★ While he does enjoy regular 69, the idea of using the Almost 69 is a bonus for him because he gets to concentrate on his own pleasure instead of trying to split his concentration between receiving pleasure and giving her oral sex at the same time.

MAKE IT HOTTER . . . If he wants her to get more out of the Almost 69 position, he can easily use his fingers to stimulate her clitoris, her g-spot, or even her anus if she likes anal play.

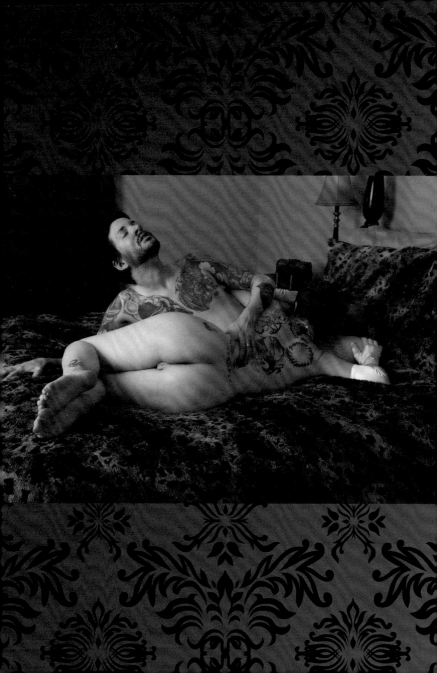

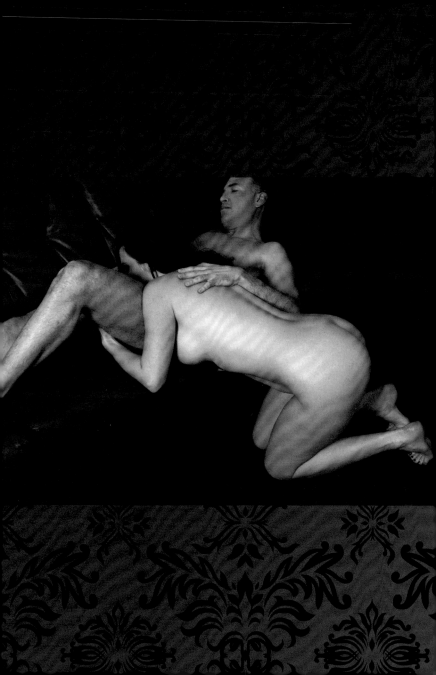

blowjob therapy

Perhaps one of the best oral sex positions for him, Blowjob Therapy allows a man to lie back, relax, and enjoy a blowjob in the utmost comfort.

HOW TO DO IT He's laid back on the sofa or the edge of the bed, relaxed and comfortable. His female partner is kneeling at his groin, leaning over the sofa or bed to perform oral sex on him. It's a fairly easy oral sex position to use, and it is much more conducive to the male orgasm than a standing oral sex position, since it can sometimes be difficult for men to ejaculate when they're concentrating on standing and not falling backwards if their knees get weak.

WHERE TO DO IT This is a perfect position for the sofa, a lounge chair by the pool, or even the edge of a low bed.

PROPS YOU'LL NEED Pillows under her knees will make it far more enjoyable for her.

DIFFICULTY LEVEL ★★★★★

HER O-METER ★★★★★ This oral sex position is fairly comfortable for the female partner and does reduce neck cramps somewhat, which can be a huge problem when it comes to giving great head.

HIS O-METER ★★★★★ What's there for a man not to love about Blowjob Therapy? He can lay back and concentrate on the pleasure with his eyes closed, or he can prop his head up on a pillow if he wants to watch the action.

MAKE IT HOTTER . . . Ladies, if you reach down and fondle yourself while you're giving your man oral sex in this position, he'll love it. He may not be able to see exactly what you're doing, but he'll really get off on the fact that you're so turned on by going down on him that you can't help but touch yourself! If he's game, this is a great position for a little prostate stimulation to really give him an explosive orgasm!

deep throat

The Deep Throat is definitely a favorite for guys because it creates some of the deepest oral penetration they've ever had during a blowjob!

HOW TO DO IT The female partner lies on the bed in such a way that her head is draped over the edge of the bed, facing up towards the ceiling. Her partner then kneels and crouches in a way that allows him to penetrate her mouth, resting his weight and controlling his movements with his arms on the bed. The Deep Throat allows her throat to be elongated so he can penetrate deeply, and it also helps her suppress her gag reflex.

WHERE TO DO IT The bed is the best place for the Deep Throat!

PROPS YOU'LL NEED None.

DIFFICULTY LEVEL ★☆☆☆☆

HER O-METER ★☆☆☆☆ If she likes being submissive, the Deep Throat will be one of her favorite ways to give her lover a blowjob. If she prefers to be more in control during oral sex, she's not going to like that he is in complete control of how fast and deep he thrusts into her throat.

HIS O-METER ★★★★★ He absolutely loves the Deep Throat. It affords him the deepest oral penetration possible, and allows his penis to be stimulated orally from shaft to tip. He also loves being in control, but he's got to watch how deep and fast he thrusts.

WARNING: A safe gesture is probably a good idea here, so she can easily and quickly let him know if he's hurting her or making her uncomfortable in any way.

MAKE IT HOTTER . . . She can reach down and stimulate her clitoris with either her hands or a sex toy. He'll love the idea that she's so turned on that she can't help herself, and he'll also love being able to look at both himself penetrating her mouth and her stimulating herself to orgasm.

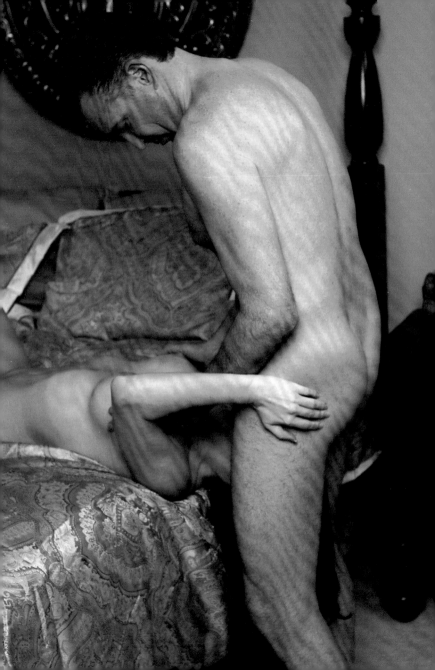

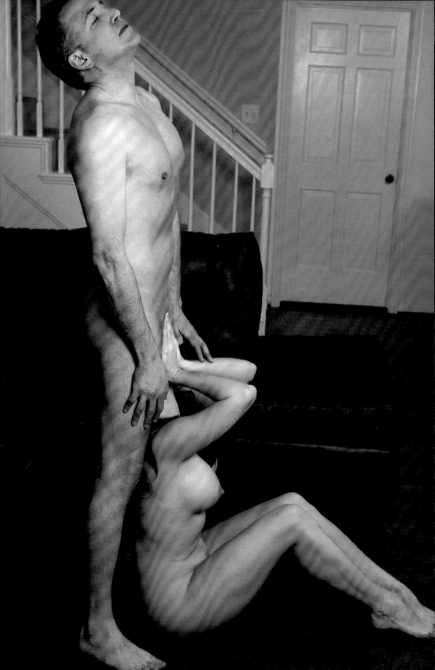

The Downward Stroke is a fun and exciting oral sex position that combines a hand job and a blowjob in a way that is comfortable for both him and her. This is a must try!

HOW TO DO IT The male partner stands with his feet a little wider than shoulder width apart, enough for her to get in between his legs to perform fellatio. The female partner sits on the ground in front of him, facing away from him, and then leans back enough so that her head and mouth are in a good position for oral penetration. She will use her hand to guide his penis into her mouth and also to stroke the base of his shaft while she sucks on the head. He can also move up and down by bending his knees.

WHERE TO DO IT The Downward Stroke is an easy one to use on the go, simply because all it requires is for the guy to drop his drawers. So for a quickie blowjob in the bathroom or in the closet at a friend's house during a party, this sex position is great. Of course, it's also good for home use and still fun if you're completely naked.

PROPS YOU'LL NEED None.

DIFFICULTY LEVEL ★★★★

HER O-METER ★★★★ The Downward Stroke is simple for her to get into, but it's bound to give her quite the crick in the neck.

HIS O-METER ★★★★ He loves the combination of oral and manual stimulation in the Downward Stroke! This is a great one for guys who have trouble reaching orgasm during oral sex alone, because the heavier stimulation can bring them to climax much more easily and quickly.

> MAKE IT HOTTER . . . She can use her other hand to stimulate her clitoris or to use a sex toy, which will give him an awesome show to enjoy while she's performing oral sex!

face straddle for him

The Face Straddle for Him is a primal, sexy way for her to submit during oral sex. He loves how animalistic this sex position is!

HOW TO DO IT The male partner gets on all fours, and the female partner lies down on her back with her knees bent and her feet flat with her head underneath her partner's hips. This allows him to bend down slightly and penetrate her mouth and throat with his penis from above. She can grasp his hips and buttocks and pull herself up to him or pull him down to her.

WHERE TO DO IT Due to the amount of space required by this position, it is much easier to do this on a bed. However, it can be done on the sofa or floor, but it isn't as comfortable.

PROPS YOU'LL NEED A pillow under her head will not only make her more comfortable, but it will lift her head and neck some to help her reach him without having to strain so much.

DIFFICULTY LEVEL ★★★★

HER O-METER ★★★★ The Face Straddle for Him may be one of her favorites if she likes for him to have control of the thrusting during a blowjob, but if she doesn't, she won't like it very much. If he thrusts too fast or too hard, it may be uncomfortable or painful for her, and she may have difficulty breathing.

WARNING: A safe gesture in this case is an exceptionally good idea, so she can quickly and easily let him know if he needs to stop because he's making her uncomfortable or she can't breathe very well.

HIS O-METER ★★★★★ He enjoys how submissive his partner is in this position and how in control he is over the thrusting. He also likes how "primal" it feels with him on all fours!

MAKE IT HOTTER . . . If he enjoys having his prostate stimulated, or even if he just enjoys a little anal play, she can easily reach around and use her hands to give him some naughty pleasure.

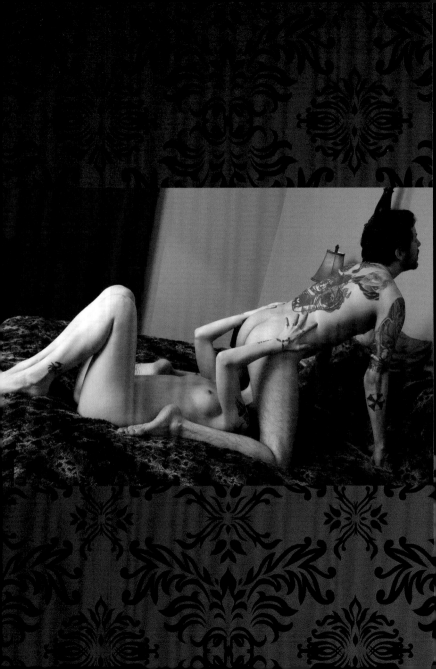

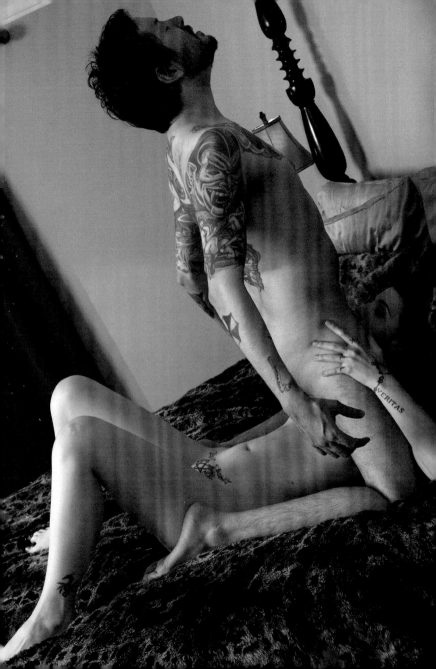

face thrust

If he likes being in control, the Face Thrust is an incredible turn on for him, but some women may find it a little uncomfortable.

HOW TO DO IT The female partner lies on her back with her head propped up by a pillow. The male partner straddles her chest on his knees, bringing his penis close to her face. He can grasp her head and use it to help him thrust in and out of her mouth. The female partner does very little in the Face Thrust oral sex position.

WHERE TO DO IT A bed is surely to be the most comfortable place for this sex position; however, it can be done on the sofa or even on the floor if her head has enough support.

PROPS YOU'LL NEED You'll need one or two pillows under her head and neck for support, and to raise her head enough for penetration.

DIFFICULTY LEVEL ★☆☆☆☆

HER O-METER ★☆☆☆☆ It's easy to get a neck cramp in this position, and since her partner is in total control, she has no say over how fast she gives him head or how deep the thrusting goes. This can easily lead to gagging and difficulty breathing.

WARNING: It's a good idea to develop a safe gesture she can use to let him know if he's getting too freaky, or if she's uncomfortable in any way. Both partners need to agree that if the safe gesture is used, the action stops immediately.

HIS O-METER ★★★★ Most guys love the idea of being in total control of a blowjob, even if they don't get to actually do it very often.

MAKE IT HOTTER . . . Since her hands are free, she can use them to caress his lower back and buttocks. If he likes anal play, she can gently play with this area using her fingers, or even massage his prostate gland. Just use lots of lube first!

The Handstand is an oral sex position for him that is challenging yet very exciting if he can pull it off! This is for adventurous couples only.

HOW TO DO IT The male partner does a handstand on the floor, with his legs straight up in the air. The female partner kneels in front of him, facing his groin, so she can perform oral sex on him.

WHERE TO DO IT The Handstand is one you should try only in the safety of your home. There's a definite possibility of falling! He'll probably want to do it on the floor as he won't be able to support himself on the bed or other soft surface.

PROPS YOU'LL NEED He may want to lean with his back against the wall for more support as he's doing the handstand. She may be more comfortable with a pillow under her knees.

DIFFICULTY LEVEL ★★★★★

HER O-METER ★★★★★ She'll like the fact that it's him getting into the wacky position instead of her, because it's almost always the other way around!

HIS O-METER ★★★★★ If he can pull off the Handstand, it's pretty fun for him. The blood rush to his head can make it more pleasurable, but on the other hand, he may find it difficult to maintain a strong erection with the blood going in the opposite direction. Also, the angle of his penis is a bit unnatural, so she definitely needs to be gentle here and not go too fast.

MAKE IT HOTTER . . . Don't worry about trying to spice up the Handstand. This is plenty hot on its own if you can actually do it!

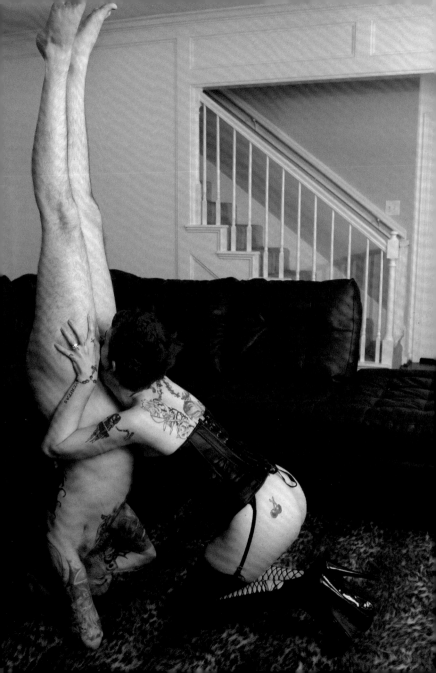

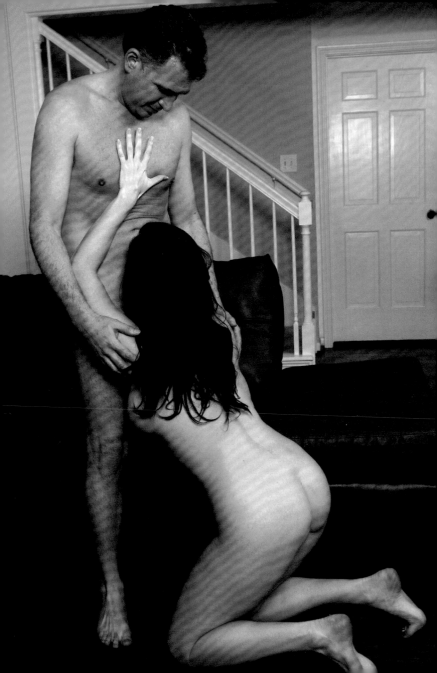

kneeling blowjob

The Kneeling Blowjob is perhaps one of the most popular oral sex positions for him, and it's definitely one of his favorites. He loves being able to look down and see her going to work on him, but if she's really good at it, she might make him weak in the knees! Keep a chair nearby!

HOW TO DO IT The Kneeling Blowjob is one of the most common oral sex positions for him. It's an extremely powerful position, and he will feel very dominant when he receives a blowjob this way. In this position, the male partner is standing and the female partner is kneeling in front of him to perform oral sex. This is a very simple yet effective oral sex position for him, although some men won't be able to orgasm well in this position because they are standing and cannot relax. Ladies, if you're good enough to make him weak in the knees, you might want to switch to a sitting oral sex position for the finish!

WHERE TO DO IT Anywhere he can stand is a good place for Kneeling Blowjob!

PROPS YOU'LL NEED She will greatly appreciate a pillow or folded blanket to slip under her knees.

DIFFICULTY LEVEL ★★★★★

HER O-METER ★★★★★ This position can help reduce neck cramps when the female partner is giving oral sex, but may be uncomfortable due to extended periods of time spent on her knees.

HIS O-METER ★★★★★ He loves getting head this way because it makes him feel very manly, as though the female partner is submitting to him—and in a way, she is. He'll enjoy looking down and watching his lover give him oral sex, and making eye contact with her when she looks up after doing her job.

MAKE IT HOTTER . . . This is an excellent "quickie blowjob" oral sex position. He can drop his drawers almost anywhere at any time, and if there's enough privacy (and even if there isn't) she can suck him off quickly. It's a standard oral sex position that you can make very, very naughty if you get creative!

peek-a-boo

An interesting twist on oral sex for him, the Peek-a-Boo is something fun to try when you want something different, but not too exotic.

HOW TO DO IT The male partner lies on his side on the bed, and his partner lies perpendicular to him, with the majority of her body behind him. He spreads his legs slightly and she brings her head up to his groin from behind, resting the weight of her head on his inner thigh.

WHERE TO DO IT Because of the space required for the Peek-a-Boo, the bed or floor is your best bet. However, the bed is going to be infinitely more comfortable for both partners!

PROPS YOU'LL NEED A few pillows for him will help prop his head up and make him more comfortable.

DIFFICULTY LEVEL ★☆☆☆☆

HER O-METER ★☆☆☆☆ The Peek-a-Boo is a comfortable position for her to be in, and it helps prevent neck cramps. This is a big plus for her, because it means she can continue giving oral sex for a significant period of time. She also has partial control here, and if he doesn't use his hand on her head, she'll have full control of the depth and speed of penetration.

HIS O-METER ★★★☆ He enjoys the Peek-a-Boo because it allows him to grasp her head and thrust if he wants, or just lie back and enjoy the sensations! He digs looking down and seeing just her head "peeking" out from in between his legs.

MAKE IT HOTTER . . . Since her hands are free in the Peek-a-Boo position, she can easily either give him some anal stimulation, if he's into it, or reach down and stimulate herself with her fingers or a sex toy so she gets some pleasure out of it too!

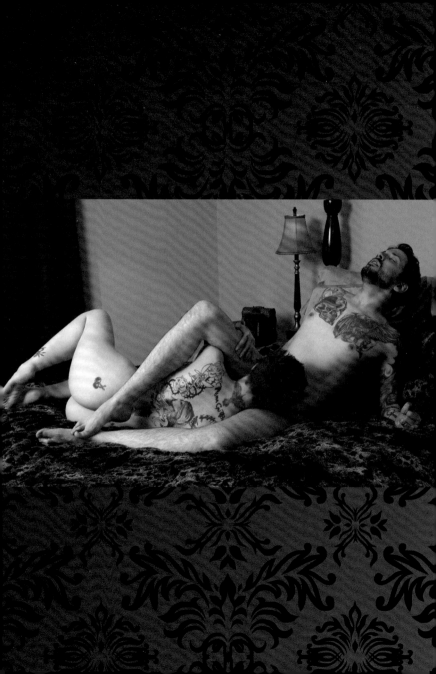

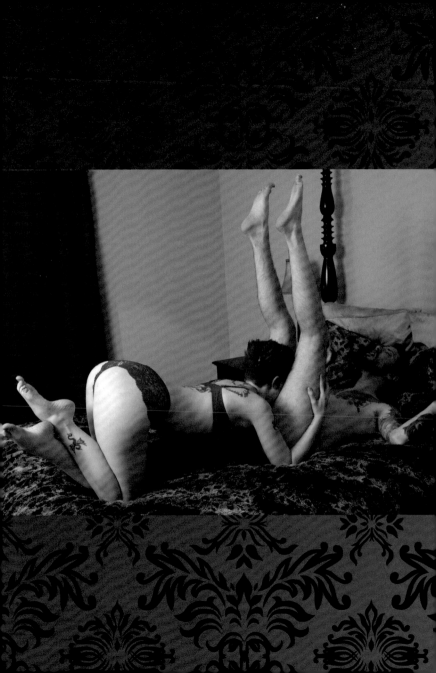

under the hood (for him)

The Under the Hood position is one that gives a man's partner full access to his nether region and makes him feel exceptionally vulnerable.

HOW TO DO IT The male partner lies on his back, and brings his legs and knees as close to his chest as possible. Typically, his legs are stretched out, but if this is difficult for him to do, a slight bend in the knees is okay. He can hold the backs of his thighs to help support his legs. The female partner then kneels to give her partner oral sex.

WHERE TO DO IT A wide space like the bed or floor is best for this position, but the bed is of course going to be much more comfortable.

PROPS YOU'LL NEED He will want a pillow under his head, and she'll want one under her knees if she's on the floor. A rolled up blanket or towel will also work.

DIFFICULTY LEVEL ★★★★★

HER O-METER ★★★★★ She likes this position because it turns the tables by giving him the opportunity to feel vulnerable and her the opportunity to be in complete control.

HIS O-METER ★★★★★ If he's not comfortable with his anal area being exposed, he's not going to like this sex position very much. However, for guys who are totally comfortable with themselves, this one is a must try! It's totally hot!

MAKE IT HOTTER . . . If he enjoys prostate massage or even a little analingus during oral sex, the Under the Hood is the perfect position to do it.

chapter 5: sitting sex positions

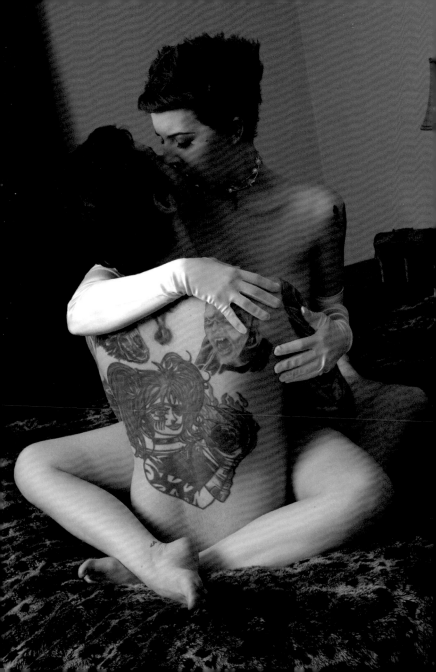

lotus

If you want to experience the utmost intimacy with your partner during sex, the Lotus is definitely the way to go.

HOW TO DO IT Both partners sit cross-legged facing each other, but the female partner will actually sit on her lover's lap with her legs wrapped around his hips so their pelvises touch. Once in position, it is more difficult to "thrust." Sex in the Lotus position involves more "rocking" than it does thrusting. This is what makes the Lotus one of the more unique sex positions that isn't as difficult to achieve!

WHERE TO DO IT Try the Lotus on the floor, bed, large rocking recliner, or anywhere you have enough space.

PROPS YOU'LL NEED If you're doing this one on the floor, you'll want a soft blanket or large pillow to prevent carpet burn!

DIFFICULTY LEVEL ★★★☆☆

HER O-METER ★★★★★ Women love the Lotus sex position! Not only does she get an extra dose of the physical and emotional intimacy she craves, the rocking and pelvic grinding does an excellent job of stimulating both her clitoris and her g-spot. This is definitely a position that she can orgasm in!

HIS O-METER ★★★★☆ If he's the sensitive type, he's going to like the emotional connection he gets out of the Lotus too. Men generally dig anything their partners are into, simply because they're psyched to have a partner who is actually enjoying herself. The rocking motion, however, will put pressure on his penis in a different way, making it feel unique and extra pleasurable for him.

MAKE IT HOTTER . . . He should give her oral sex before getting into this incredibly intimate sex position. She will literally explode on top of him!

If you have trouble with the Lotus position but still crave face-to-face intimacy, try the Assisted Lotus. It's easier and just as sensual.

HOW TO DO IT The male partner will sit in a chair with his feet on the floor. The female partner will straddle his lap while facing him and drape each of her legs over the side of the chair. She can wrap her arms around his torso for more stability during thrusting.

WHERE TO DO IT This is a great one to do in a dining room if you're alone, or any time you spot a chair without arms. It's perfect for a quickie if you don't want to get caught or a more sensual sex session.

PROPS YOU'LL NEED You can use a dining room chair or any other chair that has no arms.

DIFFICULTY LEVEL ★★★★

HER O-METER ★★★★★ There's nothing about the Assisted Lotus sex position that she doesn't like. She loves the face-to-face intimacy, she loves the comfort of doing it on a chair instead of on the bed, and she *loves* the clitoral friction. This is a very easy sex position for her to reach orgasm in, because it provides the emotional and physical stimulation she needs to climax.

HIS O-METER ★★★★★ He too enjoys the intimacy here, and although he can't thrust in and out as well as he can in other sex positions, the rocking and grinding motions that the Assisted Lotus affords are quite pleasurable. It's a great sex position for a man who doesn't want to orgasm too fast during sex and wants her to reach orgasm first.

MAKE IT HOTTER . . . Make out! Kiss and caress your lover with your mouth the entire time. Engaging this often forgotten sexual organ can really fire the Assisted Lotus up!

To take this in another direction, blindfold him and ties his hands behind the chair with a neck tie. This will awaken all of his other senses!

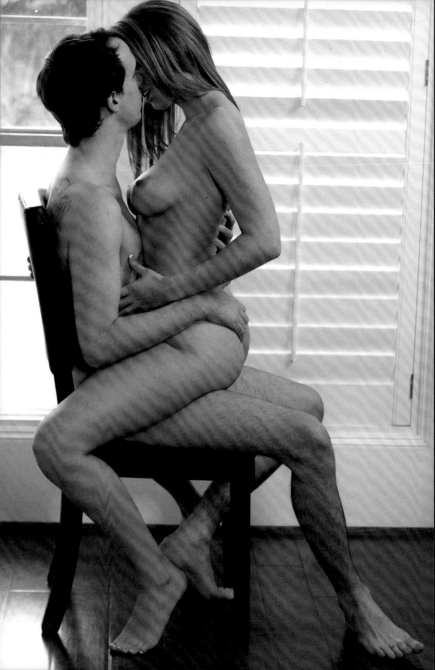

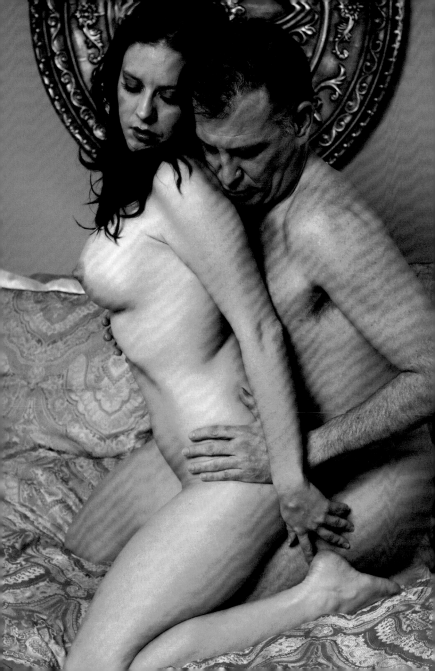

kneeling embrace

The Kneeling Embrace sex position is a sweet and sensual combination of sitting, rear entry, and woman on top that is orgasmic for both partners.

HOW TO DO IT In the Kneeling Embrace, the male partner sits on a flat surface on his knees, with his knees together or spread only slightly apart. The female partner sits in a similar manner on top of her partner's lap, facing away from him. Her knees are spread slightly to give her lover better access to her vagina.

WHERE TO DO IT While you can do the Kneeling Embrace on the floor, it's going to be hard on your knees if you choose to do so. You'll want the comfort and space of a bed or futon folded down. This could, however, be a fun sex position to try outdoors on a soft bed of grass!

PROPS YOU'LL NEED None.

DIFFICULTY LEVEL ★★★★★

HER O-METER ★★★★★ If her lover has a smaller penis, the penetration isn't going to be as deep in this sex position as others. However, she may enjoy the unique intimacy here, and the fact that he can reach around and fondle her breasts or clitoris.

HIS O-METER ★★★★★ Because his legs are pressed together, his entire penile shaft isn't going to get stimulated here, so the Kneeling Embrace may not be his favorite. However, he'll enjoy caressing and kissing his partner's back as she grinds and thrusts against him.

MAKE IT HOTTER . . . Either partner can reach forward and stimulate her clitoris for more orgasm potential for her, or if you're fairly adventurous, you might also want to try anal sex in the Kneeling Embrace sex position. This may work better for women who are new to anal sex since penetration isn't quite as deep as with other anal sex positions.

lap dance

The Lap Dance is a fun rear entry sex position, and can also be a great follow-up to a real lap dance!

HOW TO DO IT In this sex position, the male partner is seated on a surface such as the edge of the bed, sofa, or chair with his feet flat on the floor. The female partner lowers herself onto him facing away from him with her back against his chest. That sounds easy enough, but the difficult part of this sex position is getting the female partner's feet in position—her feet are tucked behind her, facing away from her on either side of her partner's body. This can be an awkward position if a woman is not very flexible.

WHERE TO DO IT A sofa, bed, or chair is best for Lap Dance, but anywhere that allows the male partner to sit on the edge with his feet on the floor will work in a pinch.

PROPS YOU'LL NEED Sofa, bed, or chair.

DIFFICULTY LEVEL ★★★★☆

HER O-METER ★☆☆☆☆ This sex position is more difficult for her to get into and stay in than her partner. It can be a little awkward, especially since the thrusting is mainly her responsibility. This is where it can get tough, because she's going to have to raise up on her shins and most women aren't used to maneuvering that way during sex. It can take some time getting used to how to move to create the best penetration.

HIS O-METER ★★★☆☆ Since he's in a natural sitting position with her facing away from him and sitting on his lap, this sex position isn't really that uncomfortable for him. He doesn't have a view, though, unless he and his lover are getting it on in front of a mirror.

MAKE IT HOTTER . . . The male partner can reach around and fondle her breasts during sex, and he can also reach down and fondle her clitoris, which is getting almost no stimulation in the Lap Dance sex position. This will make sex more enjoyable for her and increase her orgasm potential.

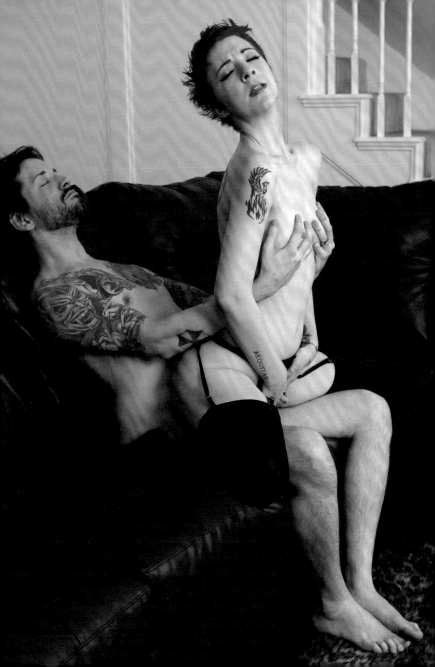

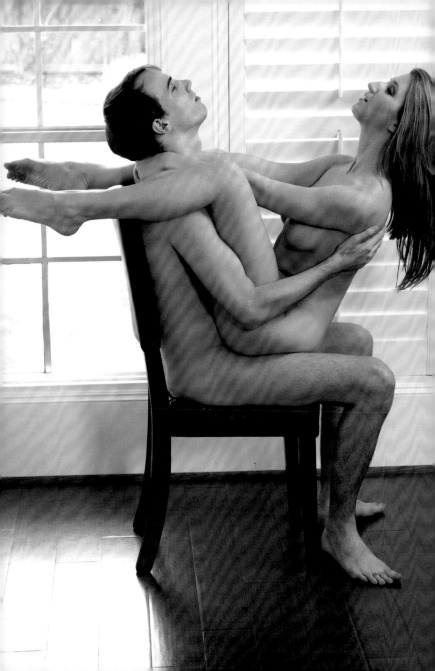

laptop

The Laptop is an interesting variation on the Assisted Lotus (see page 108), and although it looks difficult, it's really not. It's definitely a must try!

HOW TO DO IT The male partner sits in a chair with his feet flat on the floor, while his lover sits on his lap, facing him. Instead of wrapping her legs on either side of the chair, she will rest the backs of her knees on her partner's shoulders and her calves and feet on the back of the chair. She can grasp his neck to help maintain her balance, but he should be holding her lower back to help keep her steady.

WHERE TO DO IT This is an awesome sex position for a quickie at the office or anywhere else you see a chair and an opportunity!

PROPS YOU'LL NEED Almost any chair will work, but for the Laptop, you may want to use a more comfortable chair like a recliner or a nice office chair.

DIFFICULTY LEVEL ★★★★★

HER O-METER ★★★★★ She enjoys the deep penetration that the Laptop affords, because it's perfect for g-spot stimulation. Some women may need more clitoral stimulation to achieve orgasm than this position can give, but it's still a great one to try.

HIS O-METER ★★★★★ He loves the feeling of his partner's legs around his neck, and enjoys the deep penetration sensations. The Laptop is perfect for "breast guys," since he is eye level with her chest!

MAKE IT HOTTER . . . The male partner can really focus on her breasts here, caressing them with his lips and tongue. This will help her to reach orgasm even faster too!

pretzel

The Pretzel is a seated sex position that creates intimacy between both partners with its face-to-face rocking and grinding.

HOW TO DO IT To get into the Pretzel sex position, the male partner must sit on a flat surface and lie back while resting his weight on his hands behind him. His lover will then straddle him, lowering herself onto his penis. She grasps the back of her thighs and holds her legs up with her knees slightly parted so her partner can come in between them. The male partner then sits up so he is face-to-face with her. As he sits up, he will hook his legs over her legs and around her body, completing the "pretzel" configuration.

WHERE TO DO IT The bed is your best bet for the Pretzel sex position. This is a difficult position to get into and maneuver in, so you'll want the comfort and familiarity of your bed.

PROPS YOU'LL NEED None.

DIFFICULTY LEVEL ★★★★★

HER O-METER ★★★★★ She'll like the face-to-face intimacy of the Pretzel, but that's about it. This isn't going to be on her "favorites" list, and it's probably not one she'll suggest trying. She might be on board if her lover is really into exotic sex, but the penetration isn't very deep here, and her clitoris isn't adequately stimulated for her to be able to build a good orgasm.

HIS O-METER ★★★★★ He likes the novelty of this sex position, but his penis is bent at a slightly awkward angle and thrusting is fairly difficult here. It's mostly a rock and grind sort of motion. He'll want to try this move for sure because it's so exotic, but it's not going to be one he does regularly.

> **MAKE IT HOTTER . . .** Focus more on actually getting into the Pretzel sex position than on making it hotter. You're doing well if you can get in it and actually have sex for more than a few minutes!

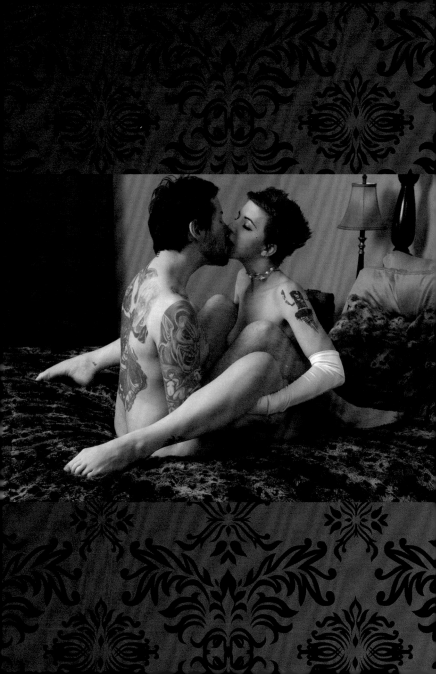

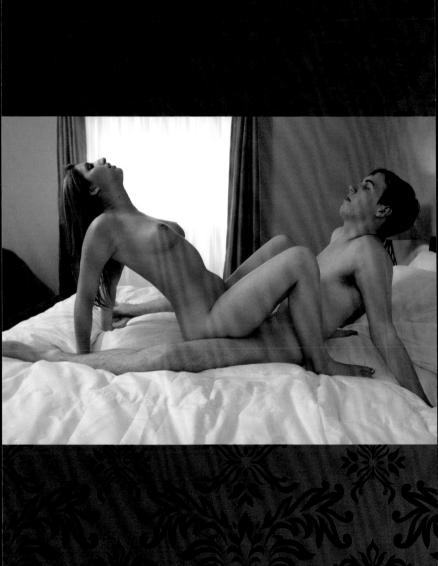

see saw

Express your intimacy and achieve intense orgasms with the See Saw. This is an easy one to do that both partners really enjoy!

HOW TO DO IT The male partner sits on the floor or the bed, with his legs stretched out and supporting his weight on his arms behind him. She straddles him, facing him, with her feet flat on either side of her lover's hips. She sits on his lap with her legs spread wide for penetration (and a great view for him!) and rests her own weight on her hands, which are behind her and grasping his ankles or shins. She does most of the work here, lifting herself up and down on his penis.

WHERE TO DO IT The bed is the most comfortable place to do the See Saw, but any wide open space (like the floor) will also do.

PROPS YOU'LL NEED None.

DIFFICULTY LEVEL ★☆☆☆☆

HER O-METER ★★★☆☆ For the See Saw to truly be effective, she must be totally and completely comfortable with her partner. Since she is open and displayed for him to see every inch of her in this sex position, she's got to be comfortable with herself as well. Confident girls will like this sex position because it gives their lovers such pleasure to see them spread out. She'll also enjoy the intimacy of being able to look him in the eye as they both experience orgasm.

HIS O-METER ★★★★★ He's comfortable in the See Saw, and he really enjoys it because he can simply sit back, relax, and watch as she grinds, rotates, and thrusts all over him. With her legs spread open, he can see everything that is happening, and that kind of visual stimulation is exactly what he needs to take a hot sex position to the next level.

MAKE IT HOTTER . . . The more she gets into the show for him, the better this position will be!

chapter 6: standing sex positions

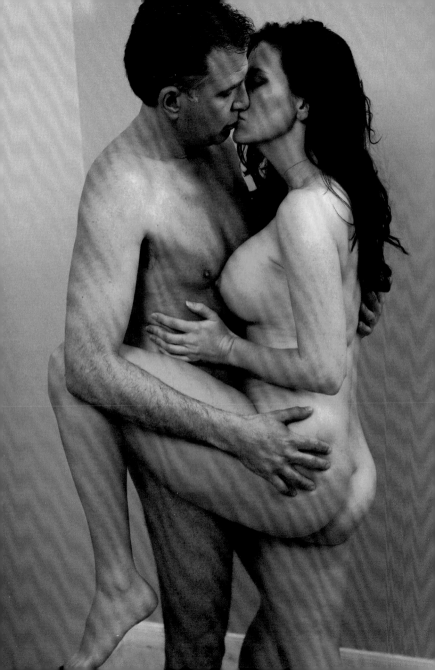

dancer

Experience incredibly hot, "I need you right now" sex with the Dancer sex position! It can be a bit difficult to master if you're not used to standing sex positions, but if you can get aligned properly, it's a super-hot yet intimate sex position to try. He feels totally in control here!

HOW TO DO IT Both partners stand facing each other (like regular Missionary only upright) and the female lifts either leg, causing her knee to bend at a ninety-degree angle. This makes it easier for the male partner to thrust while gripping her thigh or buttocks for leverage. This sex position is super sexy because it's often thought of as the "I need you now" sex position. It's as if neither of you wants to find somewhere to have sex, take your clothes off, and lie down—you want to do it right here, right now.

WHERE TO DO IT The Dancer can be done anywhere you can stand!

PROPS YOU'LL NEED A wall or chair if you're not particularly strong or don't have good balance. Leaning up against the wall can make this position more stable.

DIFFICULTY LEVEL ★★★☆☆

HER O-METER ★★★☆☆ Standing sex is hot. It's primal and conveys that he wants her now and can't wait. Women love to be wanted, craved, and desired. If he wants her so badly that he can't wait to have sex until he gets her to the bedroom, she'll be totally into it.

HIS O-METER ★★★★☆ He loves standing sex just as much. He loves feeling dominant and in control. This sex position makes him feel totally in control and very much like a man.

MAKE IT HOTTER . . . This sex position is awesome for public sex because you can do it pretty much anywhere. It's quick, it's dirty, and it's totally hot. Guys, make it even hotter by throwing your girl up against a wall (firm, but not too hard, you just want to take her by surprise). Grab her leg and hitch it up around your hips. Make it clear that you want her now, right now.

ballerina

The Ballerina is a popular standing sex position that is an excellent choice for very flexible women! Women who aren't as flexible may find this position difficult to get into and stay in, though, so if you can't hike your leg up that far, consider another position or practice stretching until you can comfortably get into the Ballerina.

HOW TO DO IT In the Ballerina, both partners are standing facing each other. The female partner raises one of her legs all the way up, resting her ankle on her lover's shoulder. Yes, she has to be incredibly flexible to do this! He holds on to her leg with one hand and her hip with the other and is responsible for the majority of the thrusting movement.

Less flexible women can simply wrap one leg around their lovers' waist (a.k.a. the Dancer sex position).

WHERE TO DO IT Standing sex positions are awesome to do in tight spaces, like when you want a quickie in the closet at a party, or are at home and don't want the kids to catch you.

PROPS YOU'LL NEED None.

DIFFICULTY LEVEL ★★★★★

HER O-METER ★★★★★ She's going to be more concerned about stretching comfortably and staying upright in the Ballerina, so she's not terribly into getting an orgasm out of it. But if she does get into it, the penetration is deep enough to elicit g-spot stimulation and possible orgasms!

HIS O-METER ★★★★★ He totally digs her leg raised like this, and if she can do the Ballerina, he'll be convinced his sex life is awesome. Guys tend to like more exotic sex positions (you know, the ones where the woman is folded up like a pretzel in a near impossible configuration), so this is high up on his "I just want to try this" list.

MAKE IT HOTTER . . . Try the Ballerina outside the house. Slip into a public bathroom stall and get it on there (just don't touch anything!), or do it in a dressing room at the department store.

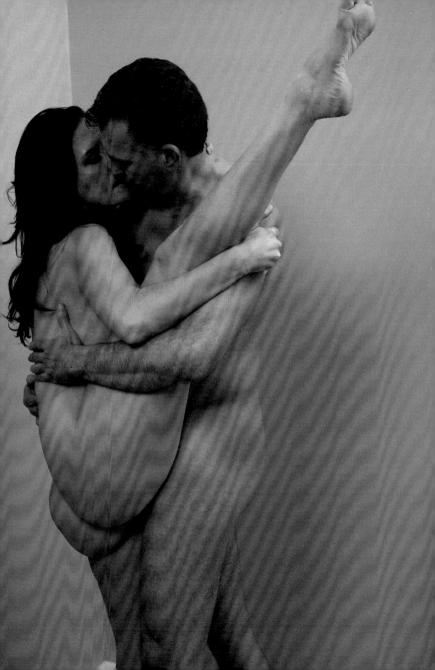

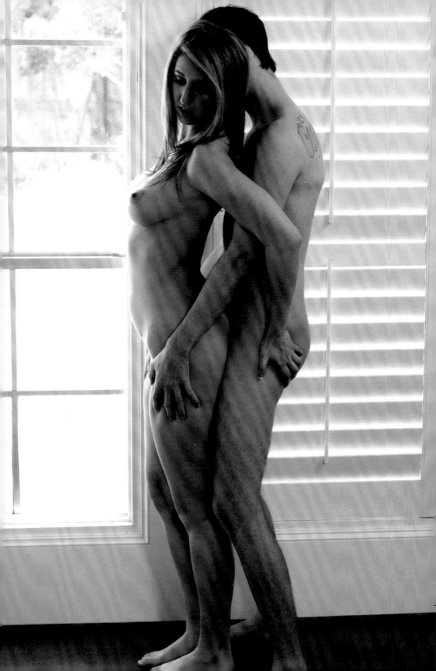

bodyguard

The Bodyguard can be extremely intimate and satisfying. He can touch her anywhere, kiss her neck, and whisper dirty things in her ear!

HOW TO DO IT The Bodyguard isn't too hard to actually get into, but it's a little difficult and awkward to keep up during thrusting. Height differences between partners can make it a little more challenging, but it's certainly not impossible. In this sex position, both partners stand, with the female partner resting her back against her lover's chest. He enters her from behind, and both partners slightly bend their knees to facilitate thrusting. It's important for the female partner to arch her back, or else he may keep "slipping out."

WHERE TO DO IT The shower, closet, or anywhere else you can stand are all great options.

PROPS YOU'LL NEED If the partners vary greatly in height, add a footstool (or stairs). This will better line up the partners' genitals for ease of thrusting.

DIFFICULTY LEVEL ★★★★★

HER O-METER ★★★★★ The Bodyguard isn't a favorite among women, unless their partners have longer penises. (Men with smaller penises who want to engage in rear entry sex are better off using the Doggy Style (see page 187) or Standing Doggy Style (see page 135), as they encourage deeper penetration.) He can make the Bodyguard better for her by reaching his hands around to her front to fondle her breasts, nipples, and clitoris.

HIS O-METER ★★★★★ He likes this position fairly well, but it's a little lackluster for him unless you're doing it in front of a mirror (which is a great idea by the way).

MAKE IT HOTTER . . . This is a great sex position to use in the shower, especially if you have a smaller shower stall.

---

piston

The Piston is a great standing position for athletic couples and allows super-deep and exotic penetration. It's definitely a must try!

HOW TO DO IT The male partner stands with his back to a chair or sofa, facing his female partner. He lifts her onto his penis (which is no small accomplishment), and she rests her feet on the surface behind him, using the leverage to help with the thrusting movements. The Piston isn't easy to do for most couples, because it requires plenty of arm strength on his part to hold almost her entire weight, and lots of leg strength on her part.

WHERE TO DO IT The piston can be done anywhere in the house where you have a surface she can rest her feet on.

PROPS YOU'LL NEED None.

DIFFICULTY LEVEL ★★★★★

HER O-METER ★★★☆☆ Although the Piston may require her to have substantial leg strength, it's worth it for all of the clitoral friction she gets. With as much effort as she is putting into the thrusting, it may be difficult for her to focus on building an orgasm, but if she's very athletic, it won't bother her a bit, and she can truly enjoy what this awesome sex position has to offer!

HIS O-METER ★★★☆☆ He likes holding her up and thrusting deeply into her, although the Piston can get quite tiring for him. If he's very fit, he'll be able to keep it up for a little while, but not necessarily long enough for both him and her to have an orgasm. This is a fun sex position to try for a little while before moving on to something more comfortable.

MAKE IT HOTTER . . . Both partners are going to be pretty occupied with supporting their weight and getting the movement down pat, so focus more on that than what you can do to "spice" this sex position up. The Piston is pretty hot in and of itself!

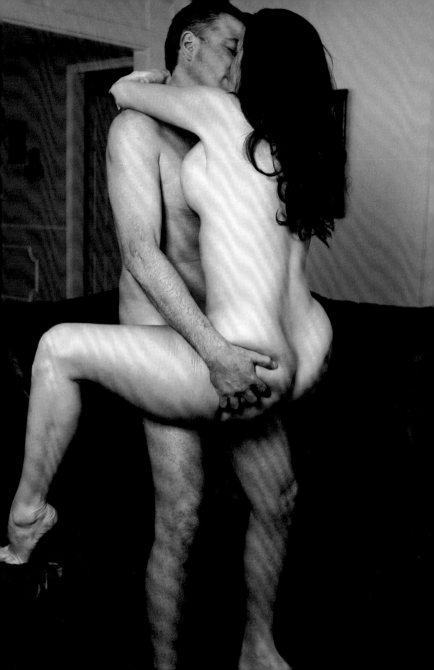

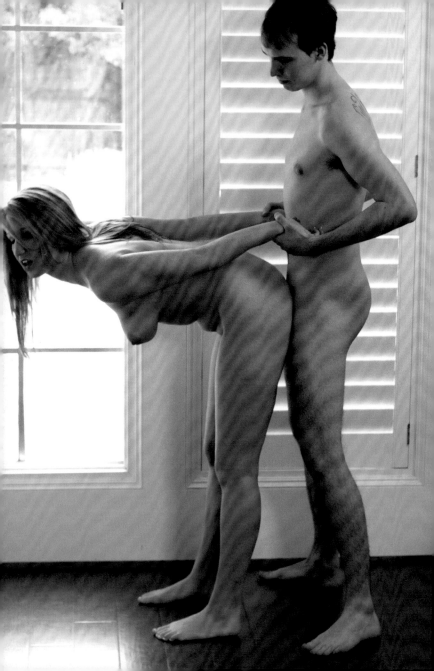

The Prison Guard is a wonderfully submissive position for the woman that allows for both vaginal rear entry intercourse and anal sex.

HOW TO DO IT The Prison Guard is a fairly easy position to get into, since both partners are standing. The female partner is standing up against her man with her back to him, and is bent over almost as far as she can go. She will bring her hands up behind her back for her partner to grasp and hold onto as he thrusts, mimicking "handcuffs" and lending the Prison Guard its name.

WHERE TO DO IT Standing sex positions are exceptionally versatile when it comes to where you can do them. You can do them in the middle of the living room, in tighter quarters like the bathroom, or even in a closet. You can do the Prison Guard almost anywhere you can stand!

PROPS YOU'LL NEED None.

DIFFICULTY LEVEL ★★★★

HER O-METER ★★★★★ If she enjoys being very submissive, she's going to love the Prison Guard. She'll also like it if she enjoys lots (and lots!) of the intense sensations that deep penetration gives. However, it's not going to be her favorite if she can only get off with more clitoral stimulation, since this sex position doesn't afford any clitoral friction at all.

HIS O-METER ★★★★★ He really enjoys the Prison Guard because it allows him complete control over his partner! She is deeply submitting to him, and not only does he get to "bind" her wrists with his hands, he gets to watch the action as he thrusts. If he enjoys being dominant, this is likely to be one of his favorite sex positions.

MAKE IT HOTTER . . . The Prison Guard can be used for really kinky, naughty anal sex but only if both partners are no strangers to anal play. This is not an anal sex position for beginners; however, it can be really hot for lovers who have done anal a few times before.

squat

The Squat is a challenging standing position that requires lots of balance on the female partner's part. It's fun to try if you can do it!

HOW TO DO IT For the male partner, the Squat sex position is particularly simple, because all he's doing is standing in front of his partner, who is facing away from him. She stands on an ottoman or stool (a chair is likely going to be too high) and squats down, bringing her buttocks close to her lover's groin. He holds on to her hips as he thrusts. The Squat is great for both rear entry and anal sex!

WHERE TO DO IT As with almost all standing sex positions, the Squat is very versatile in terms of where it can be performed. You may want to do it at home where you have access to different things for her to stand on (this will help you achieve a comfortable height), but it can be done anywhere you can stand.

PROPS YOU'LL NEED None.

DIFFICULTY LEVEL ★★★☆☆

HER O-METER ★☆☆☆☆ The Squat is more difficult for her than it is pleasurable. She may dig the deep penetration, but she may feel like she's going to fall off the stool or ottoman with the thrusting. It's also going to be very easy for her to get leg cramps in this position, even if she's quite athletic.

HIS O-METER ★★★★☆ He totally loves the Squat because it's easy for him to do and he gets to watch all the action. If he likes butts, he's really going to enjoy caressing, squeezing, and playing with her buttocks. He may be disappointed if she can't keep this sex position up for long, but it's definitely one that is difficult for her to stay in for any significant period of time.

MAKE IT HOTTER . . . If both partners are into anal play, he can easily use his hands, fingers, or a sex toy to give her anal stimulation during intercourse.

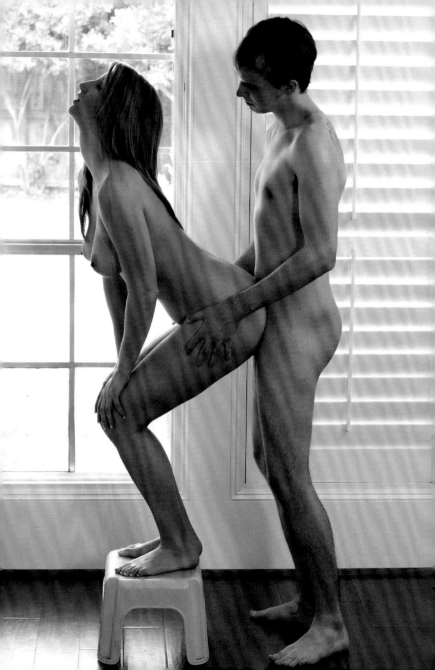

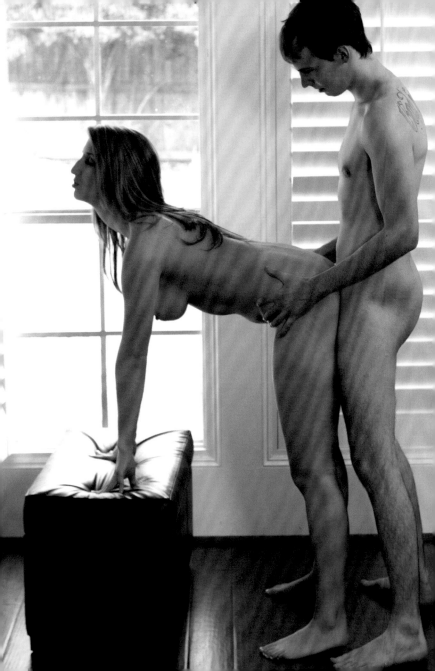

standing doggy style

Standing Doggy Style is easier on the knees than traditional Doggy Style and still provides the same perks for both female and male partners. This is another fun "animal" style sex position, because all you have to do for a quickie is pull your pants and underwear down!

HOW TO DO IT Standing Doggy Style is a little bit easier on the knees than traditional Doggy Style, mainly because both partners are standing up. This does require some kind of prop, like a chair, sofa or bed, but it's relatively simple to do. While standing, the female partner bends at the waist and places the palms of her hands on the chosen prop. The male partner enters her from behind, standing the entire time.

WHERE TO DO IT Standing Doggy can be done anywhere that she has room to bend over and support herself with her hands. Try the bed, sofa, stairs, and the hood of the car. Just use your imagination!

PROPS YOU'LL NEED None.

DIFFICULTY LEVEL ★☆☆☆☆

HER O-METER ★★★☆☆ Like traditional Doggy Style, this position is fairly good for g-spot penetration. It's much more difficult for her to reach her clitoris, however, because she's supporting the majority of her weight with her hands. She'll enjoy this position more if he reaches down and stimulates her clitoris.

HIS O-METER ★★★★☆ Standing Doggy Style provides as good a view as traditional Doggy Style, and men really dig the idea of the backdoor action, even if they're not actually getting to go in the "back door."

MAKE IT HOTTER . . . Standing Doggy Style is another one of those "got to have it now" sex positions. Both partners can drop their drawers and go at it pretty much anytime, anywhere. It's incredibly hot to want your partner so bad that you really can't even take the time to undress all the way.

chapter 7: side-by-side sex positions

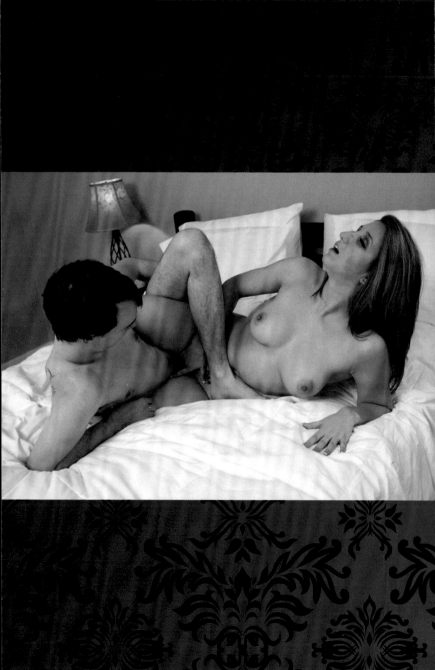

crazy starfish

For a super exotic sex position that you can add to your "we tried it" list, the Crazy Starfish is fun, yet very challenging for both partners.

HOW TO DO IT Both partners will lie on their sides facing the same way, but head to toe with each other. The female partner will lower herself onto him with her legs wrapped around his waist, and he will in turn wrap his own legs around her waist. He can brace his hands on her thighs to help facilitate thrusting, and she can support her weight with her arms behind her.

WHERE TO DO IT The bed is the best place for this one— this one requires a good deal of space. The floor works too, but carpet burns hurt! This is definitely not one you can do in a narrow space like the sofa or the backseat of a car. Too many limbs everywhere!

PROPS YOU'LL NEED None.

DIFFICULTY LEVEL ★★★★☆

HER O-METER ★★★☆☆ She doesn't have a whole lot of clitoral contact here in the Crazy Starfish, but the g-spot stimulation helps make up for it.

HIS O-METER ★★★★☆ He absolutely loves the view he gets in the Crazy Starfish, and he loves to watch the action. Bonus points for the "exotic" factor here! The only caveat for him is that his penis is bent slightly at an awkward angle, but it's likely not enough for him to be uncomfortable.

MAKE IT HOTTER . . . He can make the Crazy Starfish way hotter for her by using his hands or a sex toy to play with her clitoris. She is at a perfect angle for him to do this, so he really should do something so that both partners can get off! If she wants to give him something even more to look at, she can, of course, take matters into her own hands.

inverted spoon

The Inverted Spoon is a unique position for side-by-side fun that is a bit kinkier than traditional spooning. It's exotic, yet still intimate!

HOW TO DO IT The male partner lies down on his side on a flat surface, and his partner lies on her side facing away from him, with her back to him and with her head to his feet and her feet to his head. He can place his hands on her thighs or hips to help him thrust. This one will work a little better for most couples if they both bend at the waist just a bit. This makes for a better angle of penetration. Otherwise his penis can be at an uncomfortable angle.

WHERE TO DO IT The Inverted Spoon requires a great deal of space lengthwise, since both partners are completely stretched out. The bed is perfect for this, although the floor will work as well. If you have a futon or pull out couch, you can use that for a change in venue.

PROPS YOU'LL NEED None.

DIFFICULTY LEVEL ★★★★

HER O-METER ★★★★★ She likes the Inverted Spoon because it's easy for her lover to reach around and fondle her clitoris, or she can do it herself. She can also fondle her nipples during lovemaking, and he can, too, if he is able to reach.

HIS O-METER ★★★★★ "Butt guys" will love this sex position! It's a kinky twist on traditional spooning and is definitely one he will want to try. He likes the view and the feel of her butt grinding up against him.

MAKE IT HOTTER . . . She can raise one leg up to allow her lover to get a really nice view, although she'll need to be pretty self-confident to do this, because everything will be on display! However, this move will take the "hot" factor up a few notches. The Inverted Spoon can also be used for anal sex if both partners enjoy a little backdoor action from time to time.

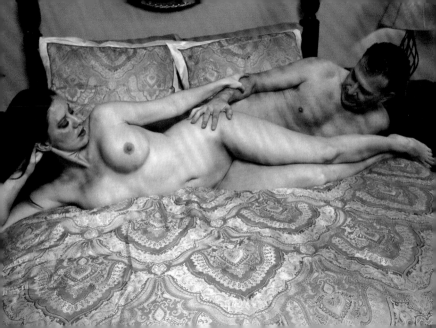

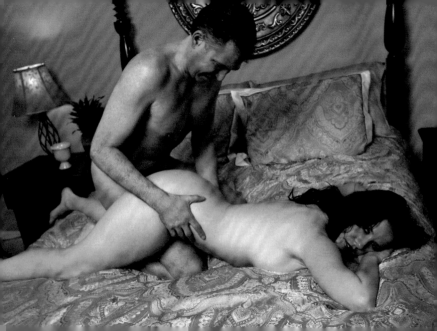

linguini

The Linguini sex position is great for deep penetration and for letting yourself go in the moment.

HOW TO DO IT The female partner lies on her side with a pillow under her head for extra support. While she lounges, the male partner kneels directly behind her butt and pushes one of his knees between her legs for insertion. The trick to this position is for the female partner to be relaxed and keep her limbs loose so that the male partner can penetrate her deeply.

WHERE TO DO IT The Linguini sex position is best performed in the bed. While the floor will work, the bed is certainly the most comfortable option. If you do decide to do it on the floor, make sure you have plenty of blankets and pillows. A soft surface is a must!

PROPS YOU'LL NEED Blankets and pillows will make sure she is relaxed and comfortable.

DIFFICULTY LEVEL ★★★★★

HER O-METER ★★★★★ She likes the Linguini sex position because she can just sit back and enjoy the ride. That, coupled with the unique angle of g-spot stimulation, can make the Linguini sex position extremely orgasmic for her!

HIS O-METER ★★★★★ This side-by-side position causes her thighs to be curved at an angle which gives him deeper access. He'll love to hear her moan as he stimulates her g-spot with ease.

MAKE IT HOTTER . . . While staying relaxed is important for the Linguini, it is critical for her to show him that she's enjoying herself as this position can tend to make her look bored if she's not actively showing her joy.

scissors

The Scissors is an exotic sex position that is easy to do and is great to use when others won't work, like during pregnancy.

HOW TO DO IT The male partner lies on his side on a bed, and lifts one of his legs so that his legs are wide open. His partner lies on her back or side perpendicular to him, straddling the leg that he has lifted so her groin is pressed against his and he is able to penetrate her. He can grasp one of her legs, and she can support her weight on her arms to help with thrusting.

WHERE TO DO IT The Scissors sex position requires so much space that you're better off doing it in the bed. While the floor will work, the bed is certainly the most comfortable option. If you do decide to do it on the floor, make sure you have plenty of blankets and pillows! It's also a fun sex position to do outdoors on a picnic blanket if you have enough privacy!

PROPS YOU'LL NEED Add some pillows for extra support here and there.

DIFFICULTY LEVEL ★★★☆☆

HER O-METER ★★★★☆ She likes the Scissors position because it's exceptionally easy for her to get clitoral stimulation. She can grind her clitoris up against his thigh, and with some lube, it can feel absolutely fantastic. That, coupled with the unique angle of g-spot stimulation, can make the Scissors position extremely orgasmic for her! Although this is an "exotic" sex position, it actually works quite well during pregnancy, when a woman isn't able to lie flat on her back in the later stages of pregnancy and can't be on top when she gets bigger.

HIS O-METER ★★★★☆ He likes being able to watch her get off in this position, and the angle of penetration makes sex feel different and new for him too. This is a great position to use if you're looking for something fairly exotic but also fairly easy!

MAKE IT HOTTER . . . This is a great position for her to reach down and stimulate her clitoris during sex either with her fingers or a good clitoral vibrator.

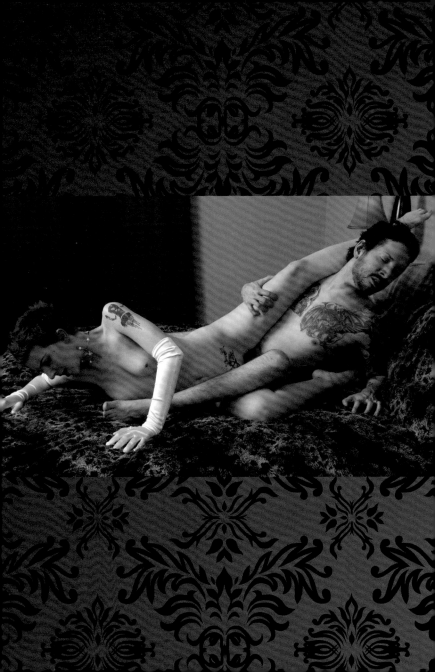

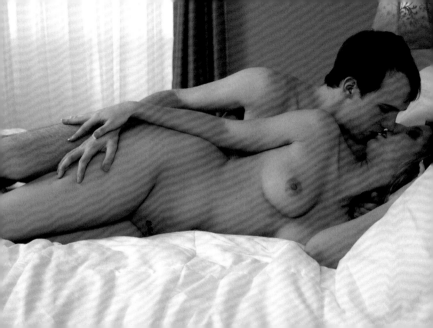

spooning

As far as romantic and intimate sex positions go, Spooning is really where it's at. Much like spooning when sleeping or cuddling, this sex position provides full body contact and plenty of opportunities for touching, hugging, kissing, and whispering in each other's ears.

HOW TO DO IT This is a wonderfully intimate sex position that will give both partners a sense of emotional connection. While both partners are lying on their sides, he enters her from behind, with his chest resting up against her back. This is very much like the "spooning" position that many couples use while sleeping, which makes this sex position so comforting and sensual.

WHERE TO DO IT The Spooning sex position works well anywhere you can snuggle such as on the sofa while watching a movie and, of course, in the bed.

PROPS YOU'LL NEED None.

DIFFICULTY LEVEL ★★★★★

HER O-METER ★★★★★ She will really enjoy the intimacy of this sex position. It feels very much like cuddling to her, which is right up her alley. The penetration might not be as deep as other sex positions. However, he can make up for this by reaching around and stroking her skin with his hands, cupping her breasts, and fondling her clitoris.

HIS O-METER ★★★★★ With this sex position, there's not much in the way for him to look at, which can be a bummer during sex. Fix this by installing a mirror next to your bed if you don't already have one. He can enter her from behind, while still getting to enjoy checking her out from top to bottom.

MAKE IT HOTTER . . . This is the perfect position for spontaneous middle-of-the-night sex. To add a BDSM twist, he can pull her hair or grab her throat from behind.

spork

The Spork is a sweetly intimate, side-by-side sex position you can use for rear entry vaginal sex or even anal sex if you like. A must try!

HOW TO DO IT Assume the traditional spooning sex position with both partners lying on their sides, and the male partner resting the front of his torso and groin against his partner's back and rear end. Instead of leaving her legs straight, as in the spooning sex position, the female partner will draw her legs all the way up against her chest so she is in the fetal position. Her partner will draw his legs up slightly to curve around her body, and will wrap his arms around her torso.

WHERE TO DO IT The bed is, of course, the easiest place to do the Spork, but feel free to get creative. Try it on a picnic blanket out in the middle of a field, or in the back of a pickup truck!

PROPS YOU'LL NEED None.

DIFFICULTY LEVEL ★★★★★

HER O-METER ★★★★★ The Spork isn't as exciting for her as other sex positions because her clitoris is almost completely non-accessible and her g-spot doesn't get much action either. This is more of a novelty for her than anything else.

HIS O-METER ★★★★★ He enjoys the intimacy of the Spork, as well as the rear entry angle. However, he doesn't get much of a view here and can't really see what is going on, so his visual system isn't going to be as stimulated as it is with other sex positions where he can watch the action.

MAKE IT HOTTER . . . She can turn her head to gaze deeply into his eyes and make a soulful, intimate connection during lovemaking. He can also reach around and fondle her breasts and nipples.

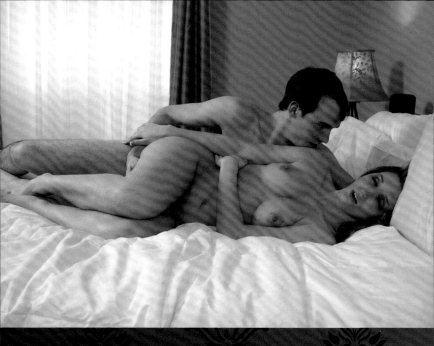

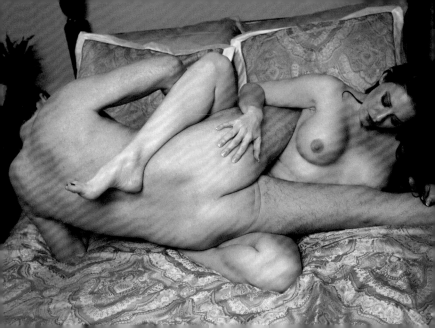

twister

If you're looking for a super-exotic sex position, the Twister should be right up your alley. Challenging, yet fun—it's a must try!

HOW TO DO IT The female partner lies on her right side, and her partner also lies on his right side, facing away from her. He will be positioned with his head to her feet and his feet to her head. Both partners will bend their left knees and lift them up, to create a space where their groins can come together to facilitate penetration. This ends up with both partners in between each other's legs. Sound complicated? It can be, but if you check out the picture on the opposite page, it may be a little easier to figure it out.

WHERE TO DO IT The bed is the best place for the Twister sex position since it requires space and is so complicated to get into. You definitely don't want to be worrying about logistics when you're busy figuring out how to thrust!

PROPS YOU'LL NEED Both partners may appreciate some pillows, but they're not necessary.

DIFFICULTY LEVEL ★ ★ ★ ★ ★

HER O-METER ★ ★ ★ ★ ☆ The Twister sex position allows her to grind her clitoris against him during penetration, increasing her orgasm potential and overall satisfaction. This may not be her favorite sex position, but it's easier for her to orgasm in this one than in many other "exotic" sex positions.

HIS O-METER ★ ★ ★ ★ ☆ The angle of penetration and the ability for him to thrust in the Twister sex position is a bit difficult for him, but he definitely likes the novelty of this one. He'll want to try it for sure, but it may not end up being his favorite either.

MAKE IT HOTTER . . . Focus on getting a rhythm down with the Twister sex position and getting more experienced at it instead of worrying about how to make it hotter. If you can accomplish this sex position and stay in it for any length of time, you're doing well!

Traditionally, the 69 is one of the most exciting ways to give and receive oral sex, because both partners get to do it at the same time. This is a great way to bring each other to simultaneous orgasm orally, and it can be a great position to use when one partner is less enthusiastic about giving oral sex.

HOW TO DO IT In the 69 the male partner lies on his back, and the female partner straddles his face, facing towards his feet. She then leans down and performs oral sex on him while simultaneously receiving it.

For the 69 to be successful, however, both partners must be clean and very comfortable with each other. Don't forget to do some basic hygiene beforehand (such as a sexy shower together), and you shouldn't have any issues.

WHERE TO DO IT You can do the 69 anywhere you can both comfortably lie down.

PROPS YOU'LL NEED None.

DIFFICULTY LEVEL ★★★★

HER O-METER ★★★★★ The 69 is a great way for a woman to receive oral sex when her partner is reluctant to go down on her without getting anything in return. The only caveat here is that she cannot fully focus on the sensations and pleasure of receiving oral sex, simply because she's trying to do two things at once.

HIS O-METER ★★★★★ Guys like the idea of being able to receive oral sex at the same time they give it, because for some men, giving oral sex isn't enjoyable in and of itself if they're not being stimulated in some way. The 69 is definitely enjoyable for him, but just slightly less enjoyable than if he were to be able to sit back, relax, and enjoy a blowjob.

MAKE IT HOTTER . . . Take your time and enjoy giving each other oral sex. Learning to move in sync and communicate sexually without speaking to each other can be extremely sexy and intimate!

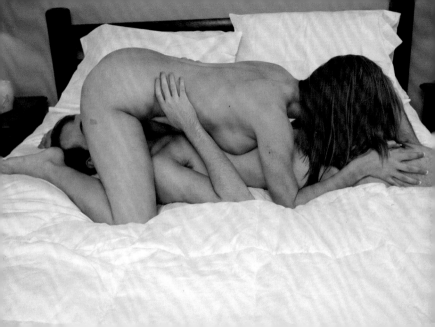

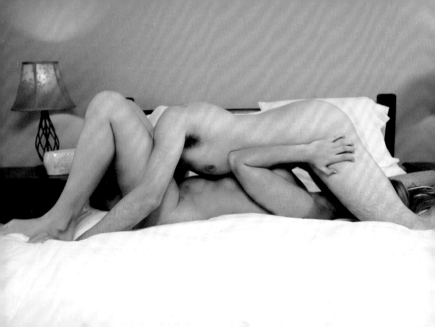

reverse 69

If the 69 sex position is one of the most exciting ways to give and receive oral sex, the Reverse 69 is a great way to switch it up.

HOW TO DO IT The Reverse 69 is a favorite among many couples because it allows both partners to give and experience oral sex simultaneously. In the Reverse 69 the female partner lies on a flat surface on her back, and the male partner straddles her face, facing towards her feet. He then leans down and performs oral sex on her while simultaneously receiving it.

WHERE TO DO IT You can do the Reverse 69 on the floor, sofa, bed, reclining chair, outdoors, or anywhere you can both comfortably lie down.

PROPS YOU'LL NEED None.

DIFFICULTY LEVEL ★★★★★

HER O-METER ★★★★★ Reverse 69 is a great way to mix it up and change positions. Just like traditional 69, it's a give and take position so both partners get to experience pleasure at the same time in this position.

HIS O-METER ★★★★★ He likes Reverse 69 just as much as traditional 69, and maybe even a little more because he has more control over the thrusting, but this position can also be a little more challenging because he will have to support his weight on his arms rather than being able to relax and enjoy the sensations.

MAKE IT HOTTER . . . Hold on tight and roll over together to switch between 69 and Reverse 69, thereby giving both partners equal time on top and bottom.

---

sideways 69

Sideways 69 is the best of both worlds.

HOW TO DO IT The Sideways 69 oral sex position is a favorite because it allows both partners to give and experience oral sex simultaneously, and no one has to be on the top or bottom. In the Sideways 69 both partners are on their sides head to toe. This can be easier on everyone's neck!

WHERE TO DO IT You can do Sideways 69 on the floor, sofa, bed, reclining chair, outdoors, or anywhere you can both comfortably lie down.

PROPS YOU'LL NEED None.

DIFFICULTY LEVEL ★☆☆☆☆

HER O-METER ★★★☆ Sideways 69 is the best of both worlds. Both partners get to relax a little, sit back, and enjoy the pleasure. She particularly likes this one because lying on her side gives her more control over both her pleasure and his level of thrusting.

HIS O-METER ★★★☆ He will enjoy Sideways 69 for the exact same reasons she does. It's less strenuous and gives him more control over his pleasure because he is free to move around more than he is during traditional 69.

MAKE IT HOTTER . . . Try adding some flavored oral sex gel to really get the most out of all of the 69 positions!

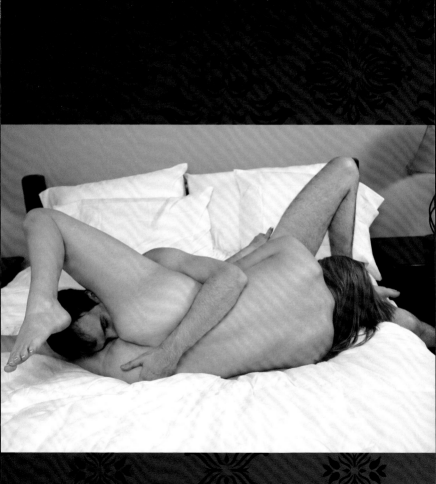

chapter 8: deep penetration sex positions

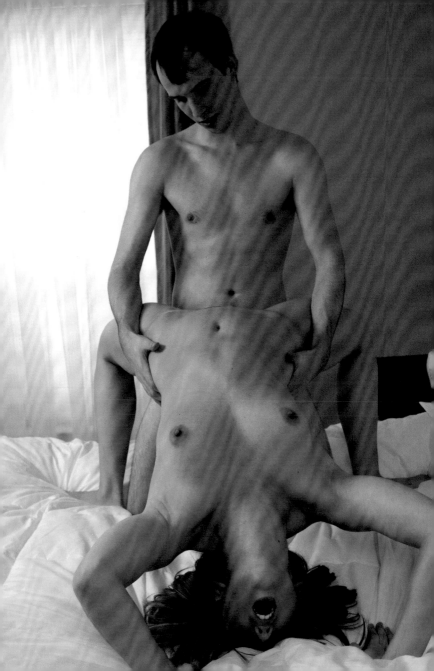

bridge

A guy will love the show a woman gives him when she bends over backwards in the Bridge sex position.

HOW TO DO IT The female partner will place her hands and feet on the floor while lying on her back and push herself up into a "bridge" position with her back arched and stomach curved towards the ceiling. The male partner kneels, aligns himself with his partner, and gently guides her hips as he thrusts. In this sex position, the female partner can lose her balance quite easily, and only very flexible women will be able to comfortably have sex in this position. However, her arched back and exposed body give him a very nice view!

If this one's too challenging, try the Cradle (see page 165).

WHERE TO DO IT The floor is excellent for this position.

PROPS YOU'LL NEED A pillow or folded towel for under his knees (rug burn hurts!). Placing an ottoman under her back for support can help her stay in this position longer.

DIFFICULTY LEVEL ★★★★★

HER O-METER ★☆☆☆☆ This can be an extremely uncomfortable sex position for a woman to get into, even if she is flexible. She may only be able to keep it up for a few minutes at a time, which is completely normal. Ladies, if you find this sex position just doesn't do it for you, don't be surprised. It's difficult! Even if you do achieve this position and can keep it up for some time, the angle of penetration doesn't provide for good clitoral or g-spot stimulation. This one's more of a novelty for your guy.

HIS O-METER ★★★☆ He will love how exotic this sex position is. It's almost as if his partner is splayed out just for his viewing enjoyment, and in a way, she is! Since she gets very little out of this sex position, it's pretty much all for him.

MAKE IT HOTTER . . . Guys, play with her nipples or rub her clitoris during the action to make it a little more enjoyable for her—and you!

climbing the flagpole

Climbing the Flagpole is a deep penetration twist on Scissors that is great for both partners. It's comfortable for most women, yet totally erotic and orgasmic! There's not too much strain on either partner as long as she is fairly flexible, and the view for both is incredible.

HOW TO DO IT   The female partner lies on her side, as though she's about to be spooned, and supports her head with her hand. The male partner straddles her leg that is resting on the bed and lifts the other so that it rests against his chest and her foot is pointed straight up towards the ceiling. To make this a bit more comfortable for her, she can add a slight bend to her knee without compromising this position at all. He will do the majority of the thrusting here.

WHERE TO DO IT   This is another sex position that requires some space if both partners are to be as comfortable as possible, so the bed or floor are good choices.

PROPS YOU'LL NEED   She will definitely want a pillow under her head if you are going to keep up the position for any length of time.

DIFFICULTY LEVEL ★★★★★

HER O-METER ★★★★★ He can grind against her clitoris fairly well in this position, making it much better for her. The deeper penetration is also good for g-spot or even a-spot orgasms!

HIS O-METER ★★★★★ He really enjoys the view in this position. He likes that she's spread wide open for him, and that he can look down and see everything that is going on. A bit more exotic than the average sex position, Climbing the Flagpole looks more difficult than it actually is. He can thrust fairly well without too much strain on his body.

> MAKE IT HOTTER . . . This is a great sex position for either him or her to reach down and play with her clitoris! This makes the Climbing the Flagpole much more satisfying for her.

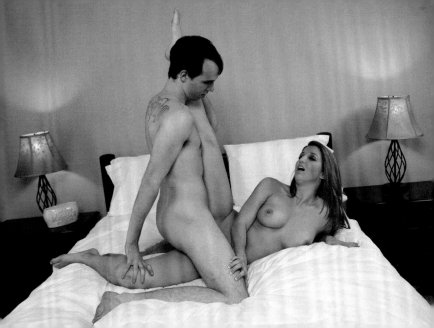

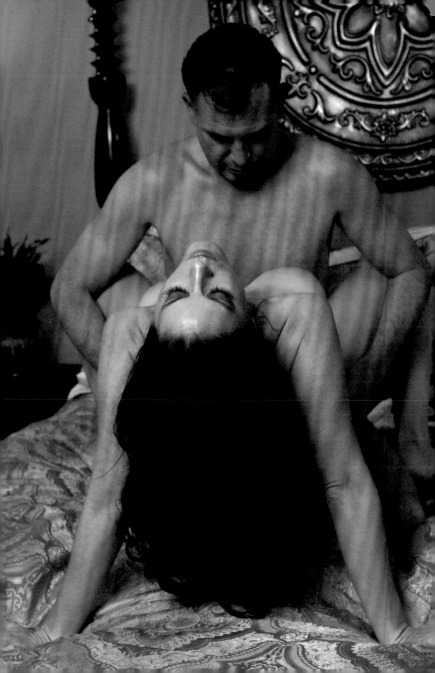

cradle

The Cradle is definitely considered an "exotic" sex position, and it can be a little difficult to master, but is highly rewarding if you do. The female partner needs to be fairly flexible, but if she can bend in this position, it gives her partner a great show and the perfect angle for nipple or clitoral play.

HOW TO DO IT The male partner kneels and rests his rear on his feet. The female partner straddles his pelvis and then bends backwards with the help of her lover's hands supporting her lower back. When the position has been achieved, it will look almost exactly like the Bridge (see page 161) but with her buttocks resting on her partner's legs instead.

WHERE TO DO IT The floor is ideal for this position, but a firm bed will work as well.

PROPS YOU'LL NEED A soft blanket or thick towel to go under his knees for comfort.

DIFFICULTY LEVEL ★★★★★

HER O-METER ★★★★★ While this sex position is a little more comfortable than the Bridge, it only allows for slightly more clitoral friction. This makes it a little easier for her to reach orgasm, but not much. With lots of foreplay beforehand, however, her partner can make sure she's turned on enough to have a better chance of reaching the big O.

HIS O-METER ★★★★★ While supporting her weight on his thighs might be a little awkward for him, the main issue here is for a man with a smaller penis. Since his thighs are pressed together, only a bigger penis will have enough length to penetrate his partner fully. If this position can be achieved well, however, he will enjoy the view. It might be a little difficult for him to thrust though.

MAKE IT HOTTER . . . Guys, spread your legs a little wider to allow your penis more room to penetrate. You might have to support your girl's hips a little more if your legs are spread, but it will be well worth it! The position will feel better to both you and your lover because of the deeper penetration and g-spot stimulation.

deck chair

The Deck Chair sex position is a deep penetration twist on Missionary that both partners will really enjoy! It's simple to do, but deeply satisfying for both partners. Get the deep sensations of Doggy Style (see page 187) or Basic Rear Entry (see page 183) with the eye contact and intimacy of the Missionary sex position.

HOW TO DO IT The Deck Chair is very similar to the Missionary, except for where the female partner places her legs. In this position, she raises her thighs to a ninety-degree angle without hooking them around his backside or resting them on his shoulders. This position is really great for g-spot or even a-spot stimulation because it facilitates much deeper penetration than the Missionary position does.

WHERE TO DO IT The Deck Chair can be done just about anywhere that you have room to lie down.

PROPS YOU'LL NEED A pillow for her lower back can make this position more comfortable, especially if you do it on the floor. It will also help tilt the pelvis for even deeper g-spot and a-spot penetration.

DIFFICULTY LEVEL ★☆☆☆☆

HER O-METER ★★★★☆ She loves this sex position because it gives her a much better angle for g-spot stimulation. It's much more likely that her partner will rub her just the right way in the Deck Chair position than in the traditional Missionary. She can spread her legs a little or a lot depending on her mood.

HIS O-METER ★★★★☆ If she gets off, he gets off. Enough said.

MAKE IT HOTTER . . . He can go up on his knees a little for more leverage and control over penetration.

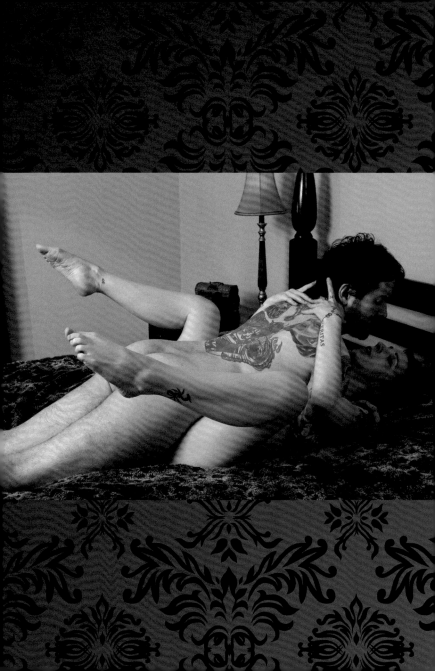

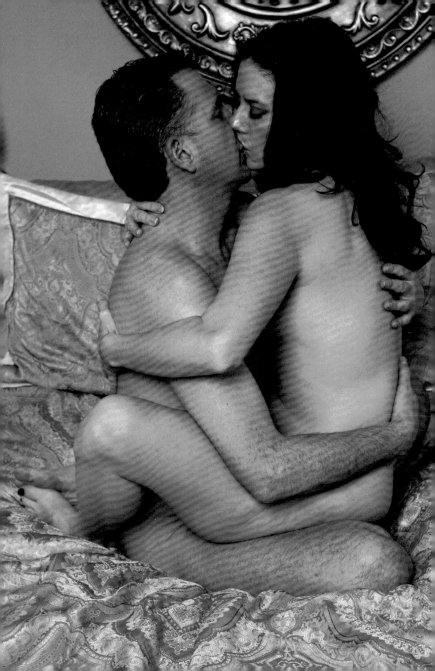

deep lotus

The Deep Lotus is an incredibly hot sitting sex position that allows for super-deep penetration and shared control between both partners.

HOW TO DO IT To get into the Deep Lotus, the man kneels on the bed or other surface and sits on his heels. His knees can be together or slightly apart. If his knees are apart, it allows for deeper penetration. The female partner faces her lover and straddles his knees, lowering herself onto him. Her knees are bent at a ninety-degree angle with her feet flat on the bed behind him. He is holding up much of her weight, but she is also providing a lot of the thrusting movement here by using her legs to lift herself up and lower herself back down.

WHERE TO DO IT The bed is definitely the best option. You're going to want the extra "bounce" the springs offer to help reduce some of the effort you have to put in with your legs.

PROPS YOU'LL NEED None.

DIFFICULTY LEVEL ★★★★★

HER O-METER ★★★★★ She likes the face-to-face intimacy of this position, and it's an excellent one for g-spot stimulation. It's also not bad for clitoral stimulation either, leading to the possibility of a blended orgasm. The only thing she doesn't like about the Deep Lotus sex position is that it requires plenty of effort, so if she's not athletic, her legs are going to cramp up pretty quickly.

HIS O-METER ★★★★★ The intimacy is great for him, too, in the Deep Lotus, but he'd much rather be watching what is going on down there, which is pretty much impossible in this sex position. However, he digs the deep penetration and the fact that she's straddling him with her legs wide open. He also enjoys the fact that this is just a touch more erotic than some of his other favorite positions.

MAKE IT HOTTER . . . Coat your bodies with a layer of baby oil so she can slide her breasts up and down during thrusting!

deep victory

The Deep Victory is an excellent sex position for g-spot and a-spot stimulation, and the face-to-face contact makes this one a must try.

HOW TO DO IT The female partner sits on a surface like a counter top or table that is roughly level with her partner's groin. He will stand and pull her legs up over his shoulders before entering her, and her feet and ankles will be resting on either side of his neck.

WHERE TO DO IT Any surface that is level with the male partner's groin will work for this position.

PROPS YOU'LL NEED If he is on the short side, or the surface you're using is on the high side, he may need a footstool to get himself up high enough to facilitate comfortable penetration. She may also want a towel, soft blanket, or pillow under her rear.

DIFFICULTY LEVEL ☆☆☆☆★

HER O-METER ★☆☆☆☆ If she's not flexible, she's not going to like the Deep Victory sex position very much at all. It will be awkward and uncomfortable for her, and she may not be able to continue in the position for very long. However, if she's an athletic girl with flexible legs, this sex position really isn't going to be that difficult for her. If you can get into this position comfortably, don't skip out on it, because the g-spot stimulation in the Deep Victory sex position is incredible!

HIS O-METER ★★★★☆ He loves this sex position because it's easy for him to get into, and it's exotic without being over the top. He can't really watch what is going on down there, but he loves the way she is spread out and waiting for him. He digs the deep penetration too, and he won't be able to last long in this position!

MAKE IT HOTTER . . . Save the Deep Victory sex position for laundry day and do it on top of the washer during the spin cycle. The vibrations will drive you both absolutely insane! Talk about hot!

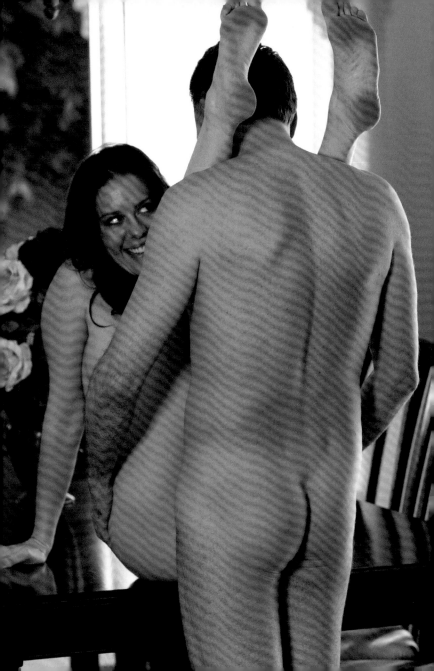

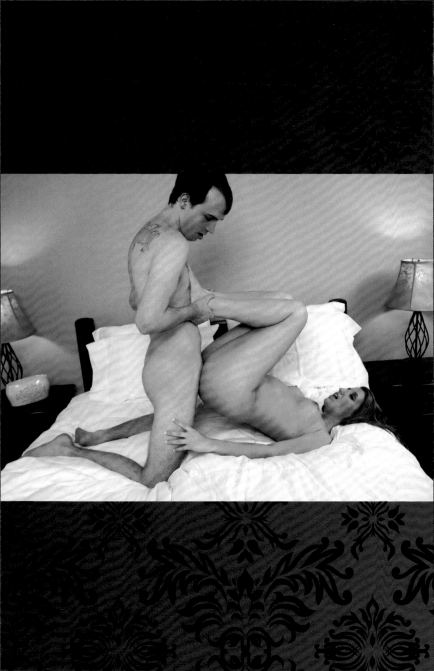

g-force

In the G-Force sex position, deep penetration is achieved in a unique way. It can be uncomfortable for the woman, but it's also really hot!

HOW TO DO IT The male partner kneels in front of the female partner who is on her back, with her knees together and drawn up towards her chest. He then lifts her hips up to meet his and enters her, with her feet either flat on his chest or in his hands. This interesting sex position can be used for either vaginal intercourse or anal sex, although it's not a good position for anal sex beginners. If you're just starting out with anal play, try another sex position first.

WHERE TO DO IT G-Force can be done on the bed, sofa, floor, or even the car if you've got a big enough back seat! Just remember that the G-Force can be rough on a woman's neck and upper back, so make sure you keep her comfort in mind.

PROPS YOU'LL NEED A liberator wedge will make it much easier to get in and stay in this position. If you're doing this position on the floor, lay down a blanket or towel first. Carpet burns hurt!

DIFFICULTY LEVEL ★★★★☆

HER O-METER ★★★☆☆ It can be a bit uncomfortable with the awkward angle created in the neck and shoulders area, but with proper support like a pillow or rolled up towel, she should be able to stay in this sex position for a decent amount of time. It definitely allows for super-deep penetration, which many women will enjoy!

HIS O-METER ★★★★★ He absolutely loves the G-Force sex position, because he gets to see pretty much everything! It's just as good as the Reverse Cowgirl (see page 49) in terms of how much he enjoys the show. The deep penetration is nice for him too, and if he gets to do anal like this, he'll be totally stoked.

> **MAKE IT HOTTER . . .** He can hold her feet in his hands to control the angle of penetration and the spread of her legs.

shoulder holder

Get the deepest possible penetration and awesome g-spot stimulation with the Shoulder Holder sex position! You really can't get any deeper than this, and the stimulation feels great for both partners.

HOW TO DO IT The Shoulder Holder is another twist on the Missionary, but it is a little more challenging. The female partner rests on her back with her legs straight up in the air, and the male partner sits up on his knees to penetrate her. Her legs will rest gently on his shoulders. This move can be a little more difficult for women who aren't as flexible in the legs. Ladies, feel free to bend your knees gently if your legs begin to feel too stretched.

WHERE TO DO IT The Shoulder Holder can be done pretty much anywhere that you can do the Missionary. Try the bed, floor, sofa, and even the recliner!

PROPS YOU'LL NEED None.

DIFFICULTY LEVEL ★★★★★

HER O-METER ★★★★★ The Shoulder Holder allows for the deepest penetration. She can fully feel him inside of her, and he can reach her a-spot easily in this position. With plenty of foreplay and clitoral stimulation, she can achieve a really intense orgasm in this position.

HIS O-METER ★★★★★ He will love the view in this sex position! It's another sex position in which he is the dominant partner, and this can be exceptionally erotic for him. He can grab her legs or hips and use them as leverage to thrust even deeper. He will really enjoy being able to feel every inch of himself inside her.

> MAKE IT HOTTER . . . To give him a super sexy view, she can spread her legs in a "V." This allows him to see and enjoy all the hot, sweaty action!

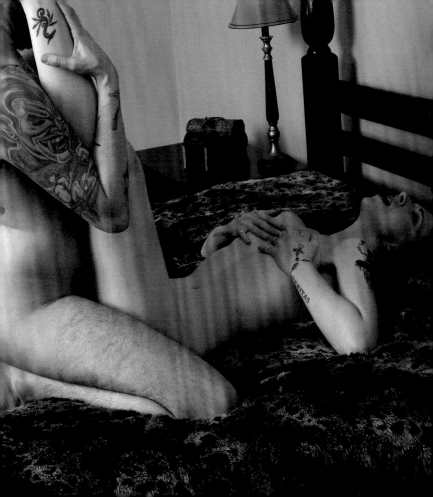

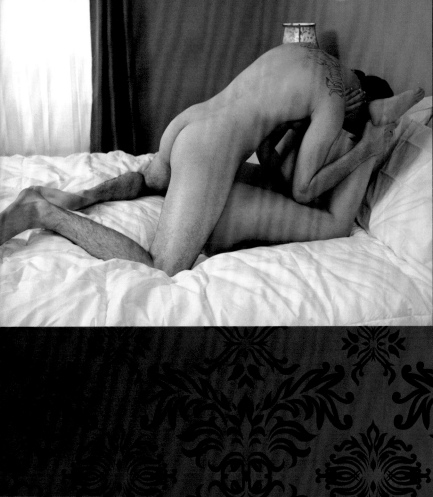

viennese oyster

The Viennese Oyster is a deliciously naughty and challenging position.

HOW TO DO IT The female partner lies on her back, raises her legs, and wraps them behind her head and crosses her ankles. Of course, this is quite a difficult position for women who aren't extremely flexible! It allows her partner to enter her quite easily because her entire groin is exposed. He should be resting his weight on his hands instead of on his partner. He can even distribute some of his weight onto his knees to make it easier on both partners.

If the female partner has trouble getting her feet to rest all the way behind her head, this position can also be achieved fairly well by simply having her partner push her legs down enough so that each ankle is on either side of her head. (This would be a modified version).

WHERE TO DO IT She needs lots of space for this one so a nice, big bed is the best choice.

PROPS YOU'LL NEED None.

DIFFICULTY LEVEL ☆☆☆☆☆

HER O-METER ★☆☆☆☆ The Viennese Oyster is going to be more difficult for her than pleasurable, unless she's very flexible, in which case the star-rating on this one goes way up! He can penetrate her deeply and the angle increases g-spot stimulation for some very intense orgasms.

HIS O-METER ★★★★☆ It's unfortunate for him that she doesn't really get off in the Viennese Oyster sex position, because he loves it. She is completely and totally spread out for his pleasure, and the feeling of his penis sliding in and out of her without her thighs or anything else getting in the way can't be beat.

> **MAKE IT HOTTER . . .** This sex position is super-hot already, and there's not much else you can do when you're occupied like this.

wheelbarrow

The Wheelbarrow is definitely a favorite for guys who enjoy exotic sex positions, even though it might not be one of *her* favorites. With him in total control, she's at his mercy! It's an excellent position for guys who really like a "butt view."

HOW TO DO IT The male partner stands normally, with his feet about shoulder width apart. The female partner will get on all fours à la Doggy Style and back up to him until she's close enough that he can bend down and pick her up from the waist. From there, he will position her hips in line with his, entering her from "behind." This requires a bit of strength on his part, but it shouldn't be too difficult. She will spread her legs out, allowing him to get a good grip on her hips and thighs to allow for thrusting. Her hands are still positioned on the floor, supporting the majority of her weight.

WHERE TO DO IT Try this one in a room with plenty of space and no furniture in the way. The Wheelbarrow definitely requires one thing, and that's space!

PROPS YOU'LL NEED She might want a towel, soft blanket, or rug to put under her hands to prevent rug burn or palm irritation.

DIFFICULTY LEVEL ★★★★☆

HER O-METER ★☆☆☆☆ There's not much in it for her as far as the Wheelbarrow goes. It's an awkward position for her to get into and for her to stay in. The blood will rush to her head, making her a little dizzy, and she may not be able to keep it up for long. However, some women who enjoy exotic positions will certainly dig the novelty here.

HIS O-METER ★★★★☆ He is in complete control sexing this position, and he loves it! The view is great, he's comfortable standing up, and it's just all around a super-hot sex position for him.

> **MAKE IT HOTTER . . .** This is a really fun position to do in a sex swing! It will give her some support and allow for more robust thrusting when both partners are not worried about falling over.

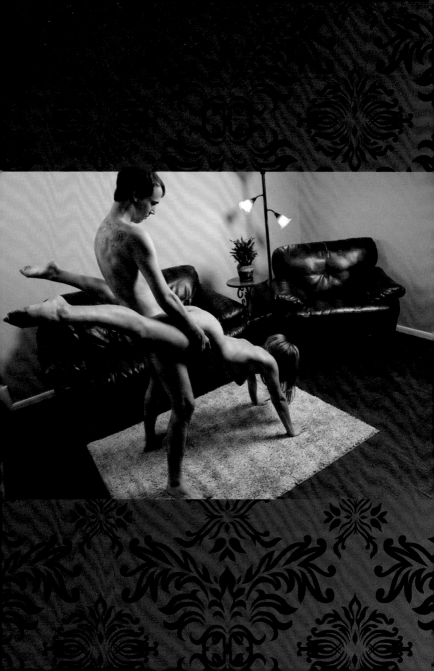

chapter 9: rear entry sex positions

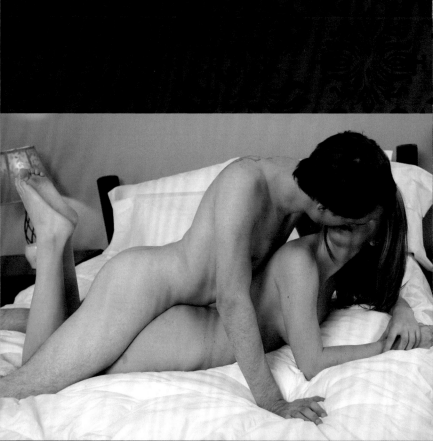

basic rear entry

This sex position is probably the easiest way to get started with rear entry, apart from Doggy Style (see page 187). When he thrusts, he can stimulate her g-spot in a unique way, and the closer her legs are together, the tighter it feels for him. This is definitely a must try!

HOW TO DO IT The female partner lies on her stomach and props her upper body up on her elbows. Her legs are slightly spread apart with her knees bent and feet in the air. The male partner approaches her from behind and drapes his pelvis over her rear so his penis can enter her vaginal opening from behind. He supports his body weight with his knees and his arms, which are positioned on either side of her upper body. The rear entry sex position can also be used for anal penetration.

WHERE TO DO IT Rear Entry can be done on the sofa, bed, floor, or any flat surface.

PROPS YOU'LL NEED A small pillow under her pelvis can raise her bottom to shorten the angle of entry for a man with a shorter penis.

DIFFICULTY LEVEL ★☆☆☆☆

HER O-METER ★★★☆☆ While rear entry does provide a unique angle to her g-spot, unless her partner's penis is on the longer side, she's not likely to get as much pleasure from this as she would if she were on top. However, if his penis is big enough, this could stimulate her g-spot in ways she's never felt before!

HIS O-METER ★★★★★ This sex position is one of the better ones for guys. The difference here is that her legs are somewhat closed and her buttocks are tight together, making her vagina feel much tighter to him. This increased friction is enough to send him over the moon!

MAKE IT HOTTER . . . Since she gets pretty much zero clitoral stimulation in this sex position, and he can't help out because he's supporting his weight on his hands, the female partner can get a lot more pleasure out of this position if she stimulates her clitoris herself either with her fingers or a small vibrator like a bullet.

The Bulldog is a unique take on Doggy Style (see page 167) that requires more leg strength from the male partner, but gives a different penetration angle.

HOW TO DO IT The female partner assumes the Doggy Style position on all fours and her partner gets behind her. Instead of resting his weight on his knees, he's actually going to crouch down with his feet on the floor or bed and bend his knees to line up his pelvis with her rear. This can require considerable strength on the male partner's part, especially during thrusting. He'll find that the angle of penetration is quite a bit different from traditional Doggy Style.

WHERE TO DO IT A flat surface is needed for both partners. She'll need to be on her hands and knees, and he will be crouched down with his weight resting on his feet. It can be done on the bed, but the male partner may be appreciative of the floor since it will allow him greater stability and balance.

PROPS YOU'LL NEED If you choose to do the Bulldog on the floor, she'll want something under her knees like a soft blanket or even a towel to prevent carpet burn.

DIFFICULTY LEVEL ★★★★★

HER O-METER ★★★★★ For women who enjoy deep penetration, g-spot stimulation (without clitoral stimulation), or anal sex, the Bulldog will be right up their alley. It's not as enjoyable for women who need a lot of clitoral stimulation to reach orgasm, but it's still a great spin on Doggy Style when you're looking for something a bit different.

HIS O-METER ★★★★★ He likes the Bulldog because the deep penetration feels awesome, but it can be difficult for him to stay crouched in that position for very long, let alone keep up the thrusting action. If he's athletic, it will be easier, but his thighs are definitely going to burn after this one!

MAKE IT HOTTER . . . If both partners can keep their balance in the Bulldog fairly well, she may be able to reach a hand down and stimulate her clitoris so she gets more out of this position too.

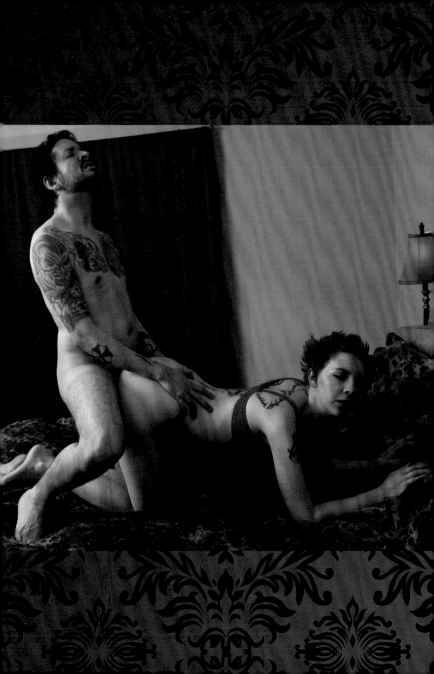

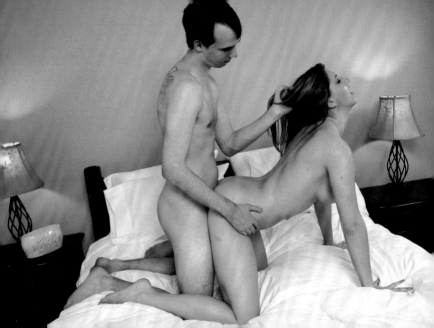

doggy style

Doggy Style is probably the most popular sex position for rear entry and for good reason! Couples love this position because of how submissive it is for the female partner, and he can watch the action while he thrusts. It's a great position for some good old-fashioned animal sex!

HOW TO DO IT The female partner gets on all fours with her weight supported on her knees and palms. Her partner approaches her from behind, holding on to her hips with his hands and supporting his weight with his knees on the floor. This is a great position for rough sex. He has more leverage with his hands on her hips and can pull her to him or push her away with his arms. It's also an excellent position for deeper penetration.

WHERE TO DO IT Try Doggy Style on the floor, bed, sofa, the bathtub/shower, or any flat surface with plenty of space.

PROPS YOU'LL NEED Both partners may need some sort of padding under the knees.

DIFFICULTY LEVEL ★★★★★

HER O-METER ★★★★★ Doggy Style is excellent for deep penetration, but not so much for g-spot stimulation. However, a woman can really get into Doggy Style if she enjoys rough sex or being dominated in this way.

HIS O-METER ★★★★★ Doggy Style is a favorite among men, simply because many men enjoy being dominant over their partners. Not to mention that he gets to stare at her backside the entire time and watch all the action!

MAKE IT HOTTER . . . A woman isn't going to get much out of the Doggy Style position unless her clitoris is being stimulated. Her partner can reach down and stimulate the clitoris or she can do it herself, either with her fingers or a vibrator. This will make Doggy Style so much better for her! To make it super naughty, the female partner can put her elbows and forearms on the floor or bed, raising her buttocks even more. Her lover will really enjoy this!

fire hydrant

The Fire Hydrant is a fun rear entry position that will bring out the animal in both partners! It's easy to do, but also super sexy. It's a simple variation on Doggy Style that mimics a dog "peeing" on a fire hydrant, hence the name. The position creates deeper penetration and gives both partners access to her clitoris.

HOW TO DO IT The Fire Hydrant starts in the traditional Doggy Style position, with her on all fours and him entering her from behind. Then she simply lifts up one of her legs and hooks it around his hip and buttock.

WHERE TO DO IT The Fire Hydrant can be done anywhere you would do Doggy Style!

PROPS YOU'LL NEED If you're not having sex on a bed or other comfortable surface, a soft blanket will protect the knees of both partners.

DIFFICULTY LEVEL ★☆☆☆☆

HER O-METER ★★★☆☆ While the Fire Hydrant sex position doesn't afford a lot of clitoral stimulation, it does provide great access to the g-spot, and even the a-spot with penetration being so deep.

HIS O-METER ★★★★☆ He loves the animalistic feel of this sex position, in which he can pull her towards him as he thrusts. He'll really like her leg hooked around him, and he can even reach down and stimulate her clitoris and labia with his hands as he gets his groove on.

MAKE IT HOTTER . . . If you have a large mirror, set it on the floor and have sex *on* it. The Fire Hydrant opens her legs up for a very nice and (ahem) not modest view of the action!

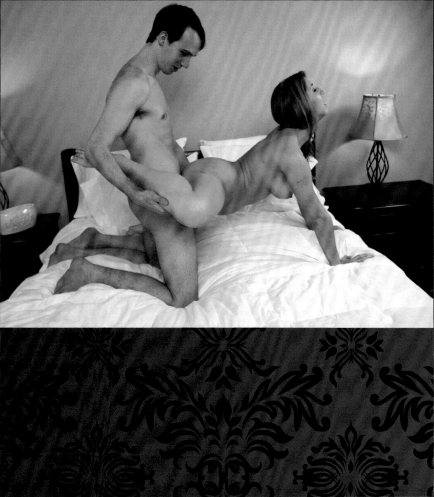

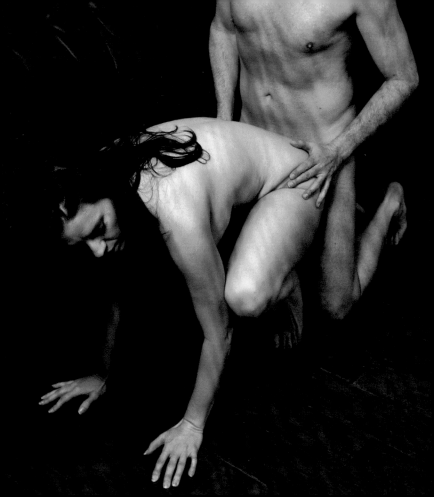

frog leap

The Frog Leap sex position is a super naughty twist on Doggy Style that gives him full access to her and facilitates super-deep penetration. It's hot!

HOW TO DO IT The Frog Leap gets its name from the way the female partner is positioned for thrusting. She is on her hands and feet with her knees bent, as though she were getting ready to play the childhood game of leap frog. The male partner sits on his knees behind her, like in traditional Doggy Style, and holds onto her hips while he thrusts. This creates deep penetration and new sensations for both partners!

WHERE TO DO IT The floor is probably the best place for the Frog Leap, simply because the female partner needs a hard surface without a lot of give to it to maintain her balance.

PROPS YOU'LL NEED He might want a pillow for his knees, and a large soft blanket is always nice when you're dealing with carpet (although carpet burns can lead to interesting conversations the next day at work).

DIFFICULTY LEVEL ★★★★

HER O-METER ★★★★ The Frog Leap is an awkward one for her to get into and stay in, unless she's on the thinner side and has a lot of strength in her legs.

HIS O-METER ★★★★★ He really enjoys the control he has in the Frog Leap, and it's comfortable for him because he isn't doing anything differently than he normally does in the Doggy Style sex position. He will also enjoy the view, especially if he prefers butts to breasts or likes anal play at all.

> **MAKE IT HOTTER . . .** Do it on the bed and have her grab on to the headboard, or on a landing with a railing that she can grab onto. This will help support her and make this move super-hot!

grasshopper

If you like exotic sex positions, the Grasshopper is definitely one you'll want to try at least want once.

HOW TO DO IT The female partner lies on her stomach with her legs stretched out. She can either lift her torso up on her arms, or she can lie her head down on a pillow if she likes. The male partner does all the work here like in the Jockey position (see page 207), but it's a little more challenging for him because of the angle of penetration. He will sit on the back of her thighs just under her buttocks and point his penis downward to enter her. His legs are open and each foot is on either side of his lover's waist, and his hands are behind him and by her feet, supporting his weight. He'll want to be very erect before attempting the Grasshopper; a soft or semi-soft penis isn't going to penetrate very well in this position.

WARNING: Go slow when trying this, and if the angle of penetration is at all uncomfortable or painful, stop immediately!

WHERE TO DO IT The bed is probably the best bet. Since you're so focused on the angle of penetration and just how to get going in this position, you don't want to add any logistical worries.

PROPS YOU'LL NEED She may want a pillow for her head if she's not holding her torso up with her arms, but it's not necessary.

DIFFICULTY LEVEL ★★★★★

HER O-METER ★★★★★ Because his penis is at an awkward angle, she won't get much g-spot stimulation. This is, however, a comfortable position for her while her lover works on his thrusting technique.

HIS O-METER ★★★★★ The odd angle of the penis in this position won't be comfortable for many men, and the thrusting action is going to be hard to figure out too. The Grasshopper is really just a novelty position to try.

> **MAKE IT HOTTER . . .** Don't worry about trying to make this sex position any hotter than it already is. You're doing well if you can get into it and actually thrust.

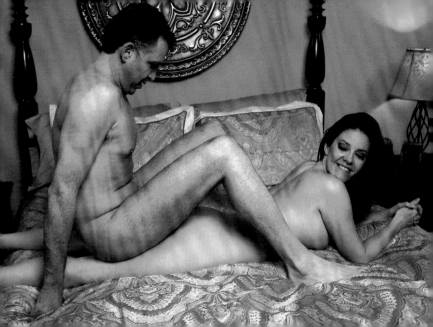

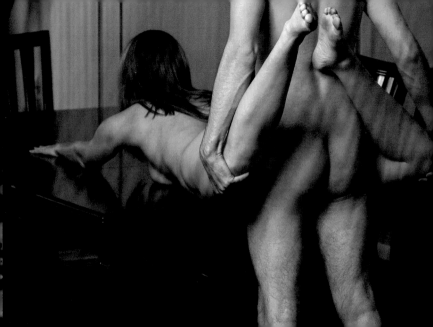

life raft

The Life Raft is a fairly easy but exciting twist on Doggy Style, and it is especially fun for the male partner. This is definitely a must try, whether it becomes one of your favorites or not.

HOW TO DO IT The female partner lays on the edge of table, desk, or bed on her belly with her knees bent and spread a little further than shoulder width apart. The male partner comes up behind her, lifting her knees and hitching them up around his hips where he can penetrate her. This may be easier to do if he penetrates first, and then wraps her legs around him. She'll continue to keep her legs wrapped around him while he thrusts.

WHERE TO DO IT The Life Raft sex position requires a bed or other surface like a desk or table that is approximately hip height.

PROPS YOU'LL NEED A blanket or thick towel is recommended if a desk or table is used. It will make this position more comfortable for her.

DIFFICULTY LEVEL ★☆☆☆☆

HER O-METER ★☆☆☆☆ The Life Raft is a position that she's not going to get much from in and of itself. She can reach her hands down and stimulate her clitoris for more pleasure during intercourse, but unless she really digs rear entry or anal sex, this is not going to be at the top of her list. It is, however, fairly comfortable for her since her lover is supporting her legs, so most women don't have a problem giving this one a try for their partners.

HIS O-METER ★★★☆☆ This is a great sex position for "butt guys," but it may get a little tiresome for him to hold her legs up and thrust at the same time. The Life Raft is still a fun one to try, because he really may like the angle of penetration and how she's spread out just for him!

MAKE IT HOTTER . . . Add a pillow or rolled up towel under her hips to enhance the angle of penetration.

---

turtle

The Turtle is an easy twist on Doggy Style that will add some spice to an old favorite. He really enjoys how submissive she is here, and how in control he is.

HOW TO DO IT The female partner rests her weight on her knees and folds over, putting her forehead as close to her knees as possible. Her breasts will be resting against the top of her thighs and she'll look almost like a turtle, hence the name. The male partner enters her from behind with his legs spread on either side of her, almost like traditional Doggy Style. It's an easy position to get into and stay in, and it's a simple twist on an old favorite if you're looking for something new to do.

WHERE TO DO IT A flat surface with a fair amount of space, such as on the floor or in the bed. The sofa or the backseat of a car wouldn't work very well for the Turtle because of the way the male partner needs to spread his legs.

PROPS YOU'LL NEED She may want a pillow under her knees or a blanket if you're on the floor.

DIFFICULTY LEVEL ★★★★

HER O-METER ★★★★ Even though there's some g-spot stimulation in the Turtle, this probably won't be a favorite sex for her. Without clitoral stimulation or even face-to-face contact, it's going to be very difficult for her to actually reach orgasm here.

HIS O-METER ★★★★★ Although this is a fun twist on Doggy Style for him and he enjoys how submissive she is in the Turtle, there's not much for him to look at here besides his lover's back. This is a fun one to try, but it's not going to be one of his all-time favorites either.

MAKE IT HOTTER . . . If you're into BDSM at all, this can be a fun sex position to incorporate some bondage into. Her hands can be bound to her ankles in this position for an ultra-submissive variation.

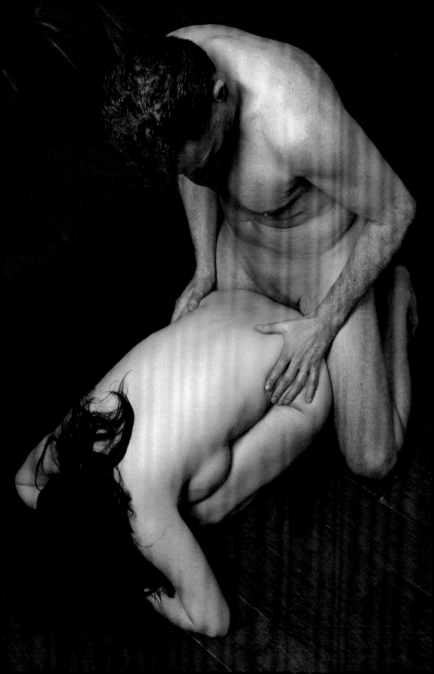

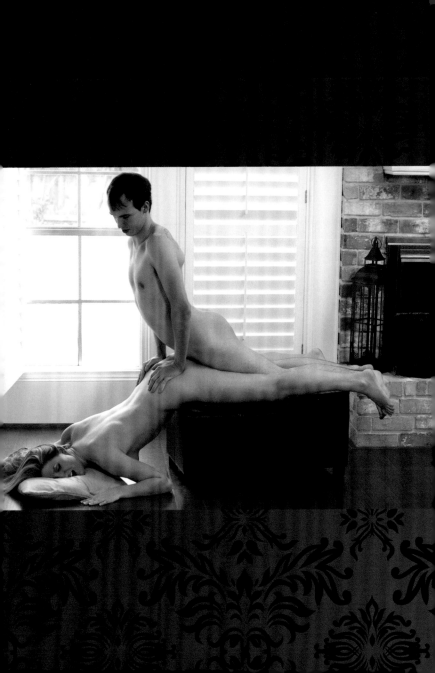

yoga master

For the athletic man, the Yoga Master is an exotic rear entry position that is a perfect fit for the super adventurous couple.

HOW TO DO IT The female partner lies on the bed on her stomach, with her hips at the edge of the bed and her torso hanging off. She rests her hands and head on the floor while he mounts her from behind on the bed. Her legs are closed and straight, and his are as well, lining up with her legs. He penetrates her from behind and uses his hands to arch his back up (almost like the Upward Facing Dog yoga move) and thrust. This is a fairly difficult position to do, but can be highly rewarding for the couple who enjoys very exotic sex.

WHERE TO DO IT This is a sex position to use on the bed (or ottoman as in the photo). You'll be using the edge of it, but it's just not one you can do anywhere else.

PROPS YOU'LL NEED She will definitely want a pillow if her head is on the floor!

DIFFICULTY LEVEL ☆☆☆☆☆

HER O-METER ★☆☆☆☆ She may not like the Yoga Master as much as he does, simply because there is very little in it for her unless she really enjoys rear entry or anal penetration. Her clitoris is well hidden and neither partner can really reach it to stimulate it. Also, because of the position of both his legs and hers, he can't penetrate her very deeply, especially if his penis is smaller. However, if she enjoys exotic positions, she will like how different this one is from others.

HIS O-METER ★☆☆★★ Although the Yoga Master is strenuous on him, he'll like how unique and exotic it is if he's adventurous. The flexible man with strong arms will likely not have much difficulty with this position, but getting the thrusting action down pat can be a bit difficult.

> **MAKE IT HOTTER . . .** Practice this one by starting with basic Rear Entry using a Liberator Wedge. He can also achieve a similar effect by standing and bending her over the back of a sofa or chair.

chapter 10: fifty shades of hot

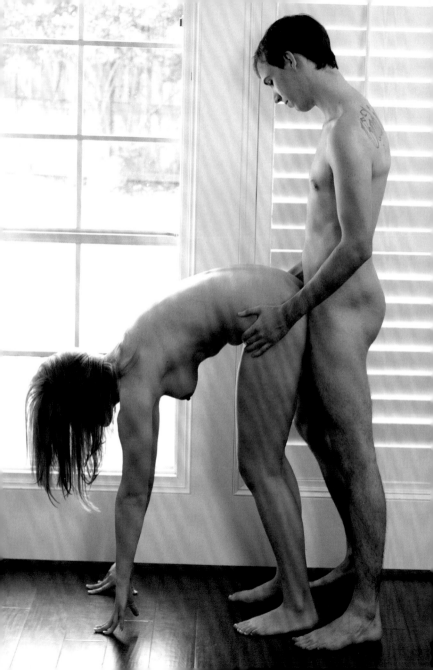

ben dover

The Ben Dover lives up to its name! She bends over and he has his way with her.

HOW TO DO IT The male partner stands with his legs slightly spread, and his partner stands in front of him with her back to him. She bends over as far as she can, with her legs as straight as possible. This is not always easy if a woman isn't flexible, so a slight bend in the knees is okay here. He will hold her hips to facilitate thrusting, going slowly at first because penetration can be quite deep in this sex position.

For couples who are very different in height, have the taller partner spread his or her legs apart until your hips are at approximately the same height. Doing this on the stairs can also help. Just make sure there is something to hold on to!

WHERE TO DO IT You don't need much space since both partners are standing, and you don't really need to be that undressed to do it! Try doing this in the department store dressing room or in the bathroom at a party.

PROPS YOU'LL NEED None.

DIFFICULTY LEVEL ★☆☆☆☆

HER O-METER ★☆☆☆☆ Although this sex position doesn't afford any clitoral stimulation, women who enjoy feeling submissive and vulnerable during sex—as well as women who enjoy very deep penetration—will add this sex position to their list of favorites.

HIS O-METER ★★★★★ He loves the feeling of control and dominance he has over his lover in the Ben Dover. He loves the view, and he loves the deep penetration. There's simply nothing about this sex position that he doesn't like!

MAKE IT HOTTER . . . The Ben Dover is a great one to use in a scenario in which the male partner is dominant. He can thrust deeply, he can talk dirty, and he can even spank her for being naughty!

boss's chair

If he wants to be in control of oral sex, this is one of the best positions to try! It's a very sexy form of submission on the female partner's part.

HOW TO DO IT The male partner sits on the edge of the sofa or bed, or in a chair, and the female partner kneels in front of him, leaning down to give him oral sex. It's an excellent position for him to be able to watch all of the action!

WHERE TO DO IT The ideal location for this one is obviously his office chair. This one is particularly hot when performed with her under his office desk!

PROPS YOU'LL NEED Add a pillow for her knees or buttocks (if she prefers to sit).

DIFFICULTY LEVEL ★★★★

HER O-METER ★★★★ If the female partner is on her knees, this oral sex position can definitely create neck cramps for her. Her neck is bent at an odd angle if she's leaning over him, and it may be difficult for her to keep up for any length of time. This can be easily remedied, however, if she simply sits cross-legged in front of him instead of on her knees. This way, her face and head are level with his genitals (depending on the height of the bed, sofa, or chair you're using) and she won't have to bend her neck as much.

HIS O-METER ★★★★★ This is another oral sex position that guys love. What men love most about this position is that they're comfortable, but they're also sitting up so they have a good view of what she's doing. Ladies, keep long hair tied back so he can actually see you suck him off. If your hair is all around your face, he might think it's Cousin It giving him head instead.

MAKE IT HOTTER . . . Ladies, let your man hold a camera (or he can use his camera phone) to video the blowjob. The Boss's Chair makes for excellent POV (point-of-view) style porn for him to fantasize about you later!

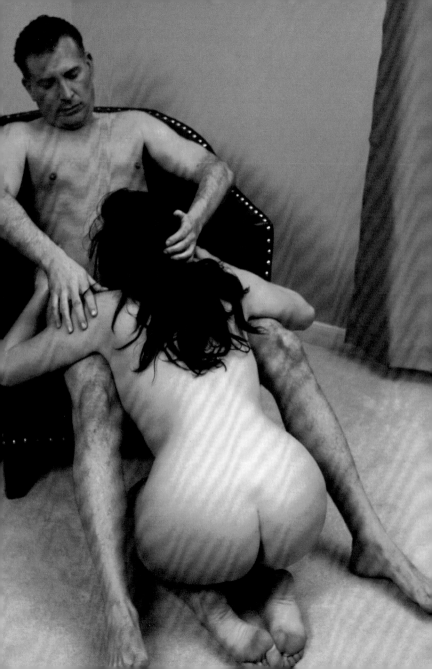

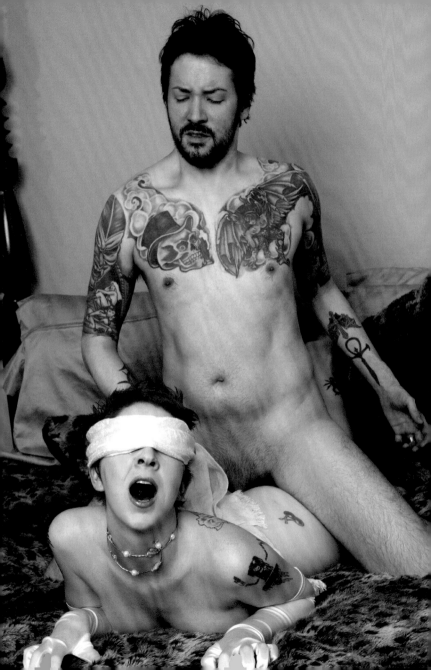

jockey

The Jockey sex position is an old favorite for both rear entry vaginal intercourse and anal sex. It's fun to do and comfortable for both partners. The position of her legs creates for a super tight entrance either way, making it hotter for both him and her.

HOW TO DO IT This is a fairly easy position to get into and is exceptionally comfortable for the female partner. All she does is lie on her stomach with her legs together, and he does the rest. He will straddle her on his knees, with one knee on either side of her hips and one hand on either side of her shoulders. This is partly why it is called the Jockey sex position; it looks kind of like a jockey riding a racehorse!

WHERE TO DO IT This is a great sex position for the bed, because it allows the female partner to be even more comfortable. But it can be done on the sofa, the floor, or anywhere else she has enough space to lie down.

PROPS YOU'LL NEED She won't mind a pillow for her head, but it's not necessary.

DIFFICULTY LEVEL ★★★★

HER O-METER ★★★★ While the Jockey is ultra-comfortable for her to get into and stay in, it really doesn't do much for her in the way of orgasms. Since she is face down, her clitoris is getting pretty much zero action, and unless she really digs rear entry vaginal intercourse or anal sex, this sex position is going to be something she does for him.

HIS O-METER ★★★★★ He enjoys being in control here, and if he's a "butt guy," he's going to like this position even more. The tightness created by her legs being pressed together is a huge plus for him, too!

> **MAKE IT HOTTER . . .** For more enjoyment on the female partner's end, she can stimulate her own clitoris during sex. This also works well (or even better!) if she's using a sex toy like a clitoral vibrator.

missionary with a twist

This is a kinky variation of the basic Missionary sex position. The twist is that her hands (and/or feet) are tied to the bed, or simply restrained in some way.

HOW TO DO IT The traditional Missionary position is often known as "Man on Top." The male partner assumes the dominant position on top of the woman, who is lying on her back. Her legs are spread enough that her lover can thrust, but they're not raised up or resting on his shoulders. While she can thrust some, the primary work done is by the man. Because the Missionary is a very passive position for the female, it doesn't take much for the man to totally dominate her mentally and physically. The dominant sensation is increased even more when her hands and feet are restrained!

WHERE TO DO IT The bed is best for this one.

PROPS YOU'LL NEED Use soft ropes or silk ties for securing her to the bed.

DIFFICULTY LEVEL ★☆☆☆☆

HER O-METER ★★★☆ Basic Missionary can be "boring" to say the least, but this "twist" really makes it hotter!

HIS O-METER ★★★★★ If he is a dominant man, he will love this. More timid men may feel overwhelmed by this one.

MAKE IT HOTTER . . . Purchase an Under the Bed Restraint System by Sportsheets to easily secure your lover whenever the desire strikes.

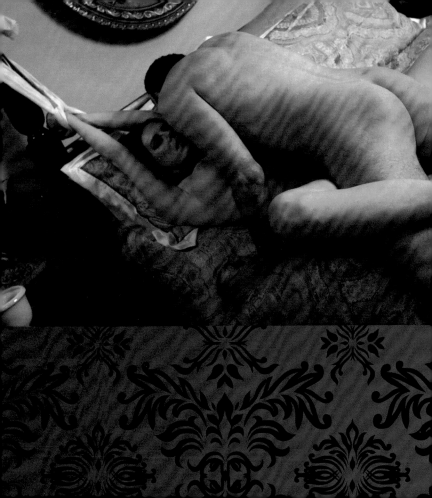

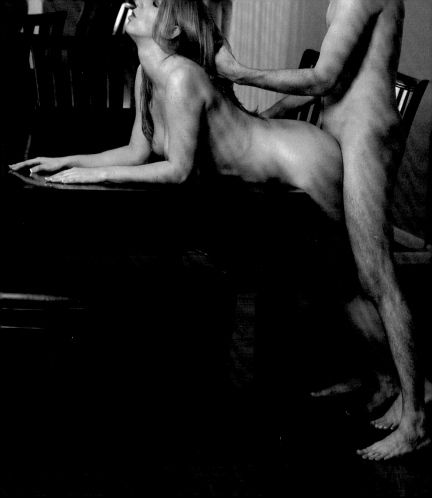

over the desk

The Over the Desk position is a kinky variation of Standing Doggy (see page 135). In this variation the female partner is bent over a desk or table and gently held down to introduce some light bondage into the position.

HOW TO DO IT The female partner stands facing away from her partner and lays flat on the desk, table, or other raised surface. He enters her from behind while standing. It's very simple but elicits exceptionally deep penetration and intense sensations for both partners.

WHERE TO DO IT Do this one anywhere you can find a flat surface for her to lay over. Tables, desks, cars, or counter tops are great options.

PROPS YOU'LL NEED In addition to the flat surface, blind-folds, cuffs, or silk ties can increase the pleasure.

DIFFICULTY LEVEL ☆★★★

HER O-METER ★★★★☆ Women who enjoy being con-trolled, really deep penetration, and a-spot stimulation will get a lot out of the Over the Desk sex position. Women who are more timid or prefer lots of clitoral stimulation during inter-course won't like this one as much.

HIS O-METER ★★★★★ He loves to control her, and he loves the Standing Doggy sex position just as much, if not more. He loves seeing her bent over just for him, and he loves grabbing her hips and thrusting deeply into her. He's in total control here, and the angle of penetration easily allows for him to insert his entire penis from tip to base. This is a must try sex position for him!

MAKE IT HOTTER . . . To increase the kink factor on this one, he can add a spreader bar to keep her legs spread wide for him!

four ways to make sex more spontaneous

FOUR WAYS TO MAKE SEX MORE SPONTANEOUS

It's easy to fall into the trap of having the same old boring sex on the same day every week, especially if you're in a long-term relationship. If you would like to take your sex life out of this rut, there are a few ways to make sex more spontaneous.

1. toss the schedule

So many couples rely on a schedule for sex that it completely downgrades their sex lives. If you know that you always have sex on Saturday morning at 8am, it's probably time to toss the schedule. A scheduled time to have sex not only hinders the excitement, it can lead to less intimacy. A relationship is a partnership and having a set day to have sex can make it seem more like a chore than a meeting of the minds. Make a conscious decision to never follow a timetable in your sex life.

2. always have condoms

One of the biggest reasons that couples can't have spontaneous sex is because of protection issues. If you're specifically trying to make your sex life more spontaneous, having the proper protection with you at all times will prevent pregnancy and the spread of STDs. This can also give you a "ready anytime" attitude with your partner. Ladies, surprise him by whipping out your own stash when the moment strikes.

3. discover each other's fantasies

When you know what turns your partner on, you can easily avoid slipping into a mundane sex rut. Make it a point to share your fantasies with each other so you can spice up your love lives with some spontaneity. You'll start to feel those butterflies when an opportunity presents itself in the blink of an eye.

Say your boyfriend has a role-playing fantasy, and you just happen to be dressed up as a sexy businesswoman. This is an excellent opportunity to take control of his desires and make your sex life a little less ordinary. When you share each other's fantasies he will also be able to take you up on a spur of the moment romp.

Say that your girlfriend has a fantasy of being taken by a mechanic. You're working on your car one day and, boom, she is instantly turned on. Share your fantasies with each other and your sex life will thrive.

4. have date nights during the week

Date nights are usually relegated to Friday or Saturday nights. Why not shake things up a bit and turn date night upside down by doing it during the week? Tuesday, Wednesday or even Monday night can give you a little something extra to look forward to when you have a spontaneous date night.

A great date night is to meet each other in a bar and pretend that you have first met. Have your partner try to pick you up for some extra spontaneity.

six hot new sex tips to try tonight

SIX HOT NEW SEX TIPS TO TRY TONIGHT

Whether you're getting tired of the same old missionary style, or you're looking to expand your already amazing sex life, the following sex tips can take you over the hump.

1. role-playing with your partner

Role-playing isn't for everybody. Plenty of men and women get embarrassed putting on costumes or improvising sexy talk. If you and your partner are comfortable with it, role-playing can be a great way to put some new kinkiness into your sex life. Some of the most common forms of role-playing involve one partner being dominant and the other being submissive.

Before you start to role play, you should always determine who is going to be dominant and who is going to be submissive. If you want to switch it up in the middle of the role-playing that is fine, too. The key is to find a healthy balance so the both of you are satisfied in the end.

2. set up barriers

This is something that is commonly found in the pick-up artist community, but it works well with couples also. Barriers are basically used to increase sexual tension. Pick-up artists use various techniques (for instance, talking dirty to a woman in a restaurant or getting her turned on in a nightclub) to increase sexual tension in an environment that cannot be used for sex.

Go out to dinner with your partner and use the barriers to your advantage. Get the sexual tension so high that you can't wait to get home.

3. switch up the dominance

There are a lot of guys and girls that love to be either dominant or submissive in the bedroom. One of the best ways that you can get out of your comfort zone and experience something different is to switch up the dominance. Instead of always having your boyfriend or girlfriend being the dominant one, take control.

If you're the one who always takes control, be submissive. In the middle of sex, switch roles so that you are either dominant or submissive. This will not only increase the sexual tension and create a really fun environment for experimentation, it can also expose you to new and creative ways of taking or letting go of control.

4. use sex toys

If you haven't tried sex toys yet, do it. Take a trip to the adult store together and pick out a small vibrator or dildo for your girlfriend. You also might want to try out a cock ring or a vibrating condom. Sex toys are there to enhance your sex life, not replace it.

So many couples think that sex toys are a form of "cheating" or "copping out." Just because you can have a really intense orgasm with a vibrator doesn't mean that your guy isn't a good lover. Try out some sex toys to get things rolling or to take your orgasms to the next level.

5. remove the anxieties

With all the pressures that come with kids, work, housework, or whatever else is going on in your life, sometimes the last thing you want to do is have sex. Remember that sex is about having fun. Try to remove some of the anxieties from your life so you can focus on your sex life.

6. double down on foreplay

Foreplay is essential for having great sex. While this is not a secret, so many men and women tend to forget it, especially when they are in a long-term relationship. Take the time that you normally spend on foreplay and double it. If you normally spend about five minutes, extend it to ten.

Mix up what you normally do so your partner is surprised. Try some kissing, then oral sex, then back to kissing or some sexy touching. This will make a big difference in turning on your partner.

about the authors

Dan and Jennifer Baritchi are the founders of AskDanAnd-Jennifer.com, which has been referred to as "Today's #1 Love & Sex Resource." AskDanAndJennifer.com has achieved a reader base of more than a million readers per month and their very successful YouTube Channel has accumulated more than sixty-five million views. Dan and Jennifer live, work, and play in Frisco, Texas.

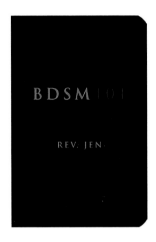

BDSM 101

by Rev. Jen

From the mind that brought you the memoirs *Elf Girl* and *Live Nude Elf* comes *BDSM 101*, a no-nonsense manual for those readers interested in learning about bondage and discipline; dominance and submission; and sadism, masochism, or sadomasochism.

For years, Rev. Jen has been coaching her readers on all sex-related matters through her articles in *Penthouse* and posts on *Nerve*, an online magazine. A self-proclaimed authority on the subject of sex (and specifically BDSM), Jen spent her early twenties working as a professional submissive at a swanky Manhattan dungeon before becoming a sex surrogate for a renowned therapist.

In *BDSM 101*, Jen shares rare insight into this oftentimes misunderstood world. Practical instructions are given on safety, communication, bondage, spanking, flogging, fetishes, humiliation, dirty talk, and more. Included are steamy, sometimes ridiculous anecdotes from Jen's past, interviews with her wacky artist friends, and basic illustrations. According to the author, "This book is what would happen if the Marquis de Sade, Andy Warhol, and Dorothy Parker got together and made a nymphomaniac bride of Frankenstein."

$16.95 Paperback • ISBN 978-1-62087-799-9

ALSO AVAILABLE

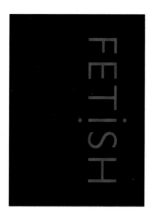

Fetish

by David Bramwell

Photographs by Petra Joy

Come and enter the sexy, seductive, and secretive world of fetish.

From agalmatophilia (the desire to have sex with a mannequin) to ophidicism (sexual arousal from snakes), this is the most comprehensive guide to outrageous erotic pleasures. *Fetish* includes stunning four-color photographs, step-by-step illustrations on acting out role-playing scenarios, and titillating advice on how to get the most out of sex toys, rubber wear, and whips. Whether you are a hard-core fetishist or simply curious, *Fetish* offers an insightful and colorful glimpse into the fascinating world of alternative sexual practices.

$14.95 Paperback • ISBN 978-1-62087-798-2

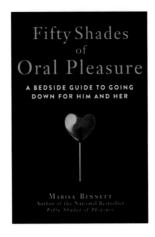

Fifty Shades of Oral Pleasure

A Bedside Guide to Going Down for Him and Her

by Marisa Bennett

In a time when taboo erotica novels are replacing the books on our coffee tables, it's no wonder that couples are exploring the naughtiest sides of sex, from silk ties and whips to candle wax and ben wa balls. But what about kink's greatest predecessor, its founding father—the blow job?

Oral sex has been one of the hottest ways to get off since the invention of the mouth, so what better way to get back to your roots and perfect your tantalizing techniques? This sexy how-to guide takes you through the Hers, His, and Us approaches to oral bliss. Get a sexy re-education on anatomy, build your oral arsenal for the most earth-shattering orgasms, bring in the kink, and try new oral positions with the help of some artfully drawn sketches. For foreplay or for your play, read some of the steamy erotica excerpts of oral sex that have been included to get you both riled and ready!

$12.95 Hardcover • ISBN 978-1-62636-089-1